THE ANCIENT TEACHING OF YOGA AND THE SPIRITUAL EVOLUTION OF MAN

AF579248

THE ANCIENT TEACHING OF YOGA AND THE SPIRITUAL EVOLUTION OF MAN

Joan Cooper

THE RESEARCH PUBLISHING CO.

52 Lincoln's Inn Fields · London

© JOAN COOPER, 1979

ISBN 0 7050 0063 X (hard-back)
ISBN 0 7050 0064 8 (paper-back)

Photoset by
Specialised Offset Services Limited, Liverpool
Printed in Great Britain for
The Research Publishing Co. (Fudge & Co. Ltd.),
Sardinia House, Sardinia Street, London WC2A 3NW.

CONTENTS

PREFACE

My introduction to yoga took place at the age of eighteen when I was studying Chinese philosophy at university and first met the Tao – or Way – and the eight-fold Path of the Buddha. Although these could not be called 'yoga' in the strict sense, they marked the beginning of an ardent desire to discover Truth, which was what following 'the way' or 'the path' meant for me. The journey from that beginning continued during the study of a variety of academic subjects in different countries, which included international law and theology and a doctoral thesis in psychology. Many experiences were to clarify and transform an eighteen-year-old's understanding before the journey led to renewed meetings with yoga teaching.

In the late fifties and early sixties I belonged to an esoteric 'school' of yoga which combined the study of ancient teachings with experience in community living. This was essentially a school of Christian yoga. The Yoga-for-Health line of development in contemporary Britain, which is largely based on traditional Hatha Yoga, only became a field for personal study in 1970.

For every stage in my personal quest for knowledge and truth I am grateful, and to every teaching upon the way I owe some debt of thanks. Each experience and every stage has been a stepping stone, but the knowledge acquired through schools or external places of learning would have brought me no nearer my own true path, and no nearer the original teaching of Yoga, if it had not been for the gradual coming into focus of the guidance and instruction I had, in fact, always been receiving from my own inner teacher.

Each person born onto this earth does have an inner teacher, but most of us are so full of our own self-will and desire that we fail even to seek the interior silence within which alone his voice can be heard. Many people end their days without awareness of the protection, inspiration, and instruction which has always been – or could always have been – theirs.

It is to my inner teacher that I owe the impetus and courage to commence both writing down and teaching the knowledge which he helped me to formulate. It is my inner teacher who reminded me of the guidelines upon which the oral teaching of Yoga was originally based and the knowledge which was transmitted by these schools of yoga down the ages. Every particle of knowledge which he clarified was imparted not through words of communication alone but also through *experience*. All that he has taught me about the essential Yoga was by way of physical, mental, and spiritual experiences. These experiences form the basis upon which the knowledge contained in this book is founded.

For nearly six thousand years the original teaching of Yoga remained an oral teaching. This oral teaching was never recorded over the long period of its history, for reasons given in the Introduction, although some of the basic knowledge found its way into certain writings – often in a different context or misrepresented. It is being recorded fully for the first time in this book because of the critical condition of life today on this planet.

Societies are being increasingly dominated in their cultural, political, and economic life by people who have no understanding of the spiritual purpose of human lives on earth. In some instances, the men ruling their societies are even dominated by the will to corrupt or destroy the spiritual substance of human life.

This teaching is being made available *now* to aid all human beings who desire spiritual growth, or who seek spiritual understanding within the confusion of contemporary life together with a re-structuring of their own lives. It is presented with the hope that in all who read it some particle of knowledge may find root, and so help to lead them to the beginning of their own 'way' to healing and wholeness.

Culbone, Porlock, Somerset
February 1979

INTRODUCTION

The Yoga* teaching which finds written expression in this book was originally an *oral* teaching and devised as such to be passed down from teacher to pupil over countless generations, without recourse to textbooks or scripture. The reason for this emphasis on a purely oral transmission of knowledge was the desire, on the part of both the originators of the teaching and also most of the subsequent teachers, to avoid any *petrification* of the teaching. Since the aim was to provide individual men (and women in later times) with knowledge concerning their spiritual evolution and to encourage the formation of a desire in them for such growth of being, written texts could have had the reverse effect by providing a structure that satisfied the logical mind but failed to stimulate the spiritual or etheric being.

The aim of the oral teaching was also to develop *flexibility* of mind and the ability in individuals to adapt to, and use for purposes of spiritual growth, the continually changing circumstances of which human life on earth is constituted in every age or epoch. To this purpose knowledge was not given as an absolute or constant *body* of data, once and for all time, but gradually and only in relation to particular men's needs at particular times. In the beginning, only an outline of purpose, certain principles, and a little knowledge about the nature of man were provided for students of Yoga. From time to time, more knowledge was given as appropriate to men's needs and *in response to* their expressed requests. This was a rule upon which the transmission of knowledge was generally based, that, apart from certain principles, it was given to men only in response to individual need or request. In this way a body of knowledge did not simply build up over the centuries to become the automatic property of later students of Yoga; but rather, at each period in history, and within each particular Yoga group or community, only certain

* Throughout this book initial capital letters have been given to those words having a clearly defined meaning for this particular yoga teaching.

aspects of the teaching were imparted which were relevant to the needs of particular individuals. No knowledge was given in order to satisfy the *logical* mind's need for order or structure or authority, or to satisfy its desire for *literal* truth; nor was knowledge provided in response to curiosity. Knowledge could only be given where there was *need*, for only then could it be used practically and not retained in the mind in abstract or theoretical form. (A written documentation of the Yoga teaching could not have contributed to the fulfilment of any of its aims and would in many respects have had an adverse effect.)

The oral teaching of Yoga – which was the first Yoga teaching – originated in the 'schools' of learning set up for this purpose in ancient Sumeria, around the beginning of the fourth millennium B.C. It originated in not one but a number of such schools, each school receiving, and working out, *part* of the knowledge about man's spiritual nature which was appropriate to that particular time and the needs of individual people at that time. Knowledge was imparted from the spiritual plane to the holy men in each school. These holy men worked out details of the knowledge which had been given to them in outline form, and the schools then brought together the different aspects of their knowledge to form a whole – but not a complete – teaching.

These holy men were 'holy' because they were *whole*[1] human beings and more highly evolved men than were those who formed the majority of people in the societies in which they lived; they were also 'holy' through the simple and single-minded desire which motivated them to serve God and man *without wanting power for themselves*.

Ancient Sumeria was the cradle of all subsequent civilisations,[2] apart from China. It was the stimulus or inspiration for all cultures to the south, north, and west. The fourth millennium B.C. saw the commencement of all historically-known civilisations in embryo, and for this reason it was the time – and the place – for the creation of a teaching which would provide guidelines for man's spiritual evolution, whatever the culture or historical epoch in which a person found himself. The oral Yoga teaching was developed and given out in the schools of ancient Sumeria and travelled on a wave of Sumerian cultural expansion as far west as that part of Britain which is now called the West Country. Here, several centres of learning were established where Yoga was taught and from which the more general cultural influence of ancient Sumeria spread. (There was no direct political influence nor any overt use of power.)

Before the fourth millennium had come to an end, however, the oral Yoga teaching was supplanted by other forms of yoga, which had, in many respects, a different aim or purpose. In the course of time, texts were compiled and students followed set and authoritative patterns of mental and physical training. Nevertheless, the oral teaching continued to exist in its original form, either openly or in secret, in many of the societies to which it had been transplanted; and it has continued down to the present day, over a period of nearly six thousand years, in the form in which it was originally presented and with the same purpose or aim.

A particular organisation of subject matter is followed in this book which may be compared with the traditional 'limbs of yoga' as expressed by the later Patanjali, nearly two thousand years ago, and by many subsequent teachers of different forms of yoga. The primary reason for this order of presentation is that it is the chronological order in which knowledge was given to students of Yoga at different historical epochs. To begin with only the material of which the first two chapters are comprised, *yama/niyama* and *asana*, was taught in the earliest Sumerian schools. Few men had at that time evolved to a stage where they could have taken in the knowledge given in subsequent chapters. The knowledge presented under the heading, *pranayama*, was taught in later Sumerian times. The knowledge comprised by the term *Pratyahara* was taught from approximately 500 B.C. onwards; and the material in the final chapter, *Dharana-Dhyana-Samadhi*, was given to students only in the Christian era, after the death of Christ.

The second and subsidiary reason for presenting the material in this particular order is that it allows for a certain amount of repetition. Facts of a psychological, etheric, or cosmic nature are often repeated in the different sections, in different contexts, so that they are seen from other perspectives. As growth of all kinds is spiral in form, each seed of knowledge is deliberately repeated in the oral teaching – but never exactly and always from a slightly different angle – so that it may take root in a person's being and grow through every stage of his learning.

It must be noted that there are gaps in the knowledge presented here. Many facts, of different kinds, can only be given orally to particular people, at particular times; they are not for general teaching, for a variety of reasons. There is also a more important reason for the omission of data or knowledge. To present the *whole* truth (if it were possible to do so), on any one of the subjects discussed in this book, would be to defeat the purpose for which the Yoga teaching was originally devised. It would deprive students of the imperative to make certain kinds of effort themselves: to develop the intuitive faculty, instead of relying on the logical mind; to learn with their *beings* rather than merely increasing the quantity of knowledge absorbed by their minds; and to bring together and work to create *for themselves* a *whole* picture out of separate or partial data. (And this effort to create a *whole* body of knowledge, as it is understood by an individual, has to be repeated at every stage in his growth of being, throughout the extent of his spiritual evolution.)

Every effort has been made deliberately to discourage the reader of this book from approaching it with his logical mind and to encourage him – or her – to make that kind of effort which results in growth of his own spiritual being. Its 'success' is only measurable in terms of individual evolution which is, in fact, not *measurable* at all.

[1]Both words come from the Old English or West Germanic *hāl* or *hālig* meaning 'whole' and 'well'.

[2]According to the oral tradition of Yoga, Sumeria was originally formed as a coherent culture and society in the mountainous region between the Black and Caspian Seas, south of what is now called the Caucasus. At a later date it extended southwards and from this centre influenced the beginnings of the Babylonian culture.

CHAPTER ONE

YAMAS AND NIYAMAS

I

The first two 'limbs' of Yoga, *yama* and *niyama*, may be considered together, for they form the ground upon which all subsequent teaching is based. This first stage in the practice of Yoga marks the commencement of personal effort, where the person endeavours to act from all that he understands – and has understood through his past experience – before he is introduced to new teaching or new knowledge.

The stage called *yama* and *niyama* states the first truth about the original Yoga teaching which is that it is about *change of being* and not simply about the acquisition of knowledge. It is about learning to act from the knowledge gained from experience – about each person learning to act from his own individual storehouse of knowledge, through which he makes it truly his own. The corollary of that first truth is that this teaching is not an abstract or theoretical philosophy but a body of knowledge about man and his spiritual evolution which is only of use if it is applied individually and acted upon. The second corollary is that learning consists in learning to act from *within* instead of from *without*: from inner discernment, inner understanding, inner truth, and not from external commandments or authority.

This first stage in Yoga may be called Karma Yoga, which means the total reversal in a man of the direction from which thinking and acting proceed. This reversal has to do with looking to the interior spiritual plane for *meaning* or *causes* or *guidance*, rather than to the external material or physical world. *Yama* or *niyama* are activities of mind in which a person seeks to discern 'right' expression from 'wrong' expression – that is, what belongs to his *own* nature as distinct from all that covers it or has been laid upon it – and to act from his inner being.

In the earliest form of Sanskrit the word *yama* meant an activity of discernment and the ability not only to distinguish right expression from wrong expression but to have control over all forms of expression that derive from *external* commands or authority. The very word *yama* stands for the essence of the original Yoga teaching about man's spiritual evolution and the importance of his becoming free from the coercion of influences external to his own nature. The teaching about *yama* states that the ability to discern right expression from wrong expression exists in the etheric (or spiritual) being of every person as a clear and actual point of reference, after the person has reached a certain stage in his own growth of being. Thus, the activity of discernment is based on a *real* point in a man's inner being, not on anything imposed from without or placed in him through auto-suggestion.[1]

The five *yamas* comprise an activity of discernment that applies to the working of a man's whole being: the attitudes of mind upon which a person bases his judging, the motives for his external forms of behaviour, the direction of his thinking, the kind of active/passive balance in his being, and the direction and use of his energy. In each case it is a matter of discerning the extent to which a particular aspect of his being derives from *within* and seeking to have command over all manifestations which derive from *without*: i.e. from forms of direct social/cultural authority or from the more subtle forms of internalised social coercion. This does *not* mean that a person should attempt to stop or directly oppose what he observes as coming from outside himself – even if this were possible. *To have command over* means to be aware of and to learn to make some effort to choose or determine the extent of the influence. This is the only time when the pupil of Yoga is asked to make efforts of this kind, because it is only through these efforts to have command over influences which have for a long time determined the structure and behaviour of his own being, that a person begins to realise something of the dangers that threaten his experience and, even more, the *growth* of his being. Through making the kind of effort called for by the *yamas* he begins to realise the amount of effort that is needed to reverse the direction in which his being has been oriented and to begin to express from within himself; he begins to understand the qualities of persistence and courage necessary to pursue the aims of the Yoga teaching.

1. *The first Yama concerns* Judging

Judging comes from man's mind and is the foundation of his activity and thought. The discernment which the *yamas* call for, and which proceeds from an actual point in a person's etheric being, is the commencement of judging.

Every manifestation of a man's being is based upon some form of assessment, some distinction as to 'this' or 'that', some judgment formed regarding the situation and persons concerned. Every decision is based on a prior judgment; every action is based on selection which is preceded by the activity of judging. All thinking proceeds by the selection of one thing and the rejection of another. The life of every man, in thought and act, depends upon how he judges and the ground from which he judges. It was to uncover this subconscious foundation of a person's life and its expressions that the first *yama* was called 'judging' and that the pupil's first efforts were directed towards becoming aware of the basis upon which his judgments were founded which determined the daily expression of his thought and action.

With growth in awareness, a person comes to see that *assessment* of people or situations often implies *censure* as well, and that this censure comes from forms of value-judgment that do not derive from his own experience. He discovers that whereas *assessment* is based on his own experience and upon a certain degree of personal involvement and understanding, *censure* is based on a feeling of separateness from the person judged. The feeling of moral superiority which it implies derives from abstract categories outside the persons involved. With growth in awareness, a man becomes increasingly sensitive to the entirely different nature of those judgments which derive from outside his own understanding and experience to the forms of judgment which are reflections of his own nature or etheric being. The first kind of judging he comes to think of as 'wrong' judging and the second as 'right' judging. Violence is implicit in all forms of wrong judging because wrong judging comes from a feeling of being separate from other people. There is no violence in right judging which derives from the etheric being of a person, however unformed or weak the nature of that being. Finally, the person discovers that the origin of the various forms of wrong judging lies in the authority-structure or value-systems of the society around him or in the home or school environments which formed his early thinking.

As awareness deepens and a person gains clearer insight into the various strata which form the basis for his judging, a desire to gain control over certain manifestations of wrong judging begins to express itself within his own etheric being. The efforts a person makes to control judging must always be the expression of his own desire if they are to be effective, for *real* effort does not derive from commandment or coercion of any kind.

In order to have command over wrong judging, a person also learns to understand more about the nature of other people and sees that they can only change from *where they are* in themselves. This quality of acceptance is one of the results that comes to a person through the efforts he makes in relation to this *yama*.

2. *The second Yama concerns* Personal Action and Social Behaviour

The discernment on which this *yama* is based has to do with identifying *social behaviour* as distinct from the *personal actions* which are expressed from the true nature of the person.[2] As in the case of *judging*, this *yama* also teaches the pupil to discern the different forms and layers of his behaviour that derive from requirements placed on him by his society in all its implicit as well as explicit forms. Just as the desire arises in a person to learn to control certain forms of *judging*, which do not belong to his etheric nature, so a similar desire eventually awakens in him to have command over those forms of behaviour which are entirely derivative and do not reflect his own nature. But the desire to *take command* only grows through observation and understanding.

There are 'wills' within each person that do in fact attract and desire many forms of Social Behaviour. These cannot be stopped at command, and this *yama* – like all the *yamas* – is about inner discernment and becoming more aware of the nature and origin of all that the being of the person expresses. As awareness grows, so a little control becomes possible in the form of choice.

Personal Action, as opposed to Social Behaviour, does not mean 'right' or 'moral' action. Personal Action is action which expresses from the etheric being of the person, and each person's etheric being contains weaknesses as well as strengths. The actions which express from weaknesses – for example, the actions which are caused by fear – are 'right' actions for that person only in so far as they are a reflection of his true nature. A man's etheric being is visible to himself only by way of reflection, in the actions it expresses. Only in this way is the many-sidedness of his true nature revealed to himself, of which weaknesses are part. Until he begins to see himself as he is, a person cannot desire change of being.

Social Behaviour may be 'right' for the society in which a person lives. From the point of view of society, controls must be placed on the most extreme actions of its members. But unless – or until – a person is able to reveal in some degree what society seeks to hide or repress, he can never discover the true nature of his own etheric being and begin to fulfil the reason for which he came into a physical life. This is why every form of authoritarian or highly-organised society is inimical to individual spiritual evolution, because it prevents the individual person from expressing and therefore facing his true self from which experience alone comes the desire for his own spiritual growth.

Most of a person's actions may be expressive of Social Behaviour and derive from a set of *mores* imposed from outside himself by the society in which he lives. In fact, these actions derive only in part from overt social convention or ethics. Most people are a multiplicity and most actions, even without the particular social context in which they are expressed, would *not* flow naturally from their own inner beings; these actions would in some form falsify or cover up or distort the etheric being because they would reflect a texture of half-truths and fantasies which the person *believed* to be true about himself. Although most of these half-truths and fantasies derive originally, and in a certain sense, from outside the person, he weaves their particular form himself as his own protective covering with which he meets and relates to the world around him. It is this 'protective covering' which he thinks of as his 'self'; with it he seeks to impress or have power over others; because of it his feeling of 'I' or 'self' is outward-oriented and dependent upon the world in which he lives, the way it treats him, the relationships it has with him. This state of affairs is exactly opposite to the conditions in which man was originally intended to live and which are best suited to the growth of his own being.[3] Few people on earth now live so that their actions express from their own etheric beings, whatever their degree of spiritual advancement. Yet this was – and is – the aim of man's physical life on earth.

3. *The third Yama concerns* Dissatisfaction

The third *yama* is about *dissatisfaction.* The life of every person on earth today is stratified with layers of dissatisfaction or discontent; the kind and quality of life on the physical earth increases man's vulnerability to it. Dissatisfaction is the largest single drain on man's energies and is often, and in many of its forms, completely unconscious to him. It is of great importance for the Yoga pupil to become aware of the sources of dissatisfaction in himself and to make effort to control them.

The cause of every form of dissatisfaction lies in *wrong thinking.* Thinking may be defined in terms of the direction from which man thinks, 'wrong' thinking being every kind of mental activity which proceeds from the material/physical world in the form of expectations or desires. Every expectation, every anticipation that depends for its fulfilment upon material or physical results, and every desire to possess or obtain even intangible responses to request – in fact, every possible form of *wanting something*, makes a person vulnerable to dissatisfaction if the desired result is not obtained or the expectation fulfilled. To *want something* – anything – creates a dependence upon factors outside the person and often beyond his control. The desire for personal achievement – even the desire for psychological achievements – is a desire for results that are measurable by external criteria or through comparisons of a quantitative nature. Everything can be a source of dissatisfaction.

Dissatisfaction does not rest solely on desire or anticipation, but on every form of dependence which makes man vulnerable to change. *Change* is a principle upon which all physical life is based; change is continuous, even if ordered, and nowhere on earth do manifestations of life remain the same or ever return exactly to previous forms of expression. Yet most people *act* as if the world around them *ought to be* unchanging, and their thinking proceeds from static concepts or absolutes and expectations of a kind of automatic result which could only be looked for on an assembly-line. The mental world inhabited by an ever-increasing number of people is a fantasy world structured by concepts which apply to machines rather than to people and which create forms of expectation not realisable on any plane of existence.

Wrong thinking is not only thinking from the wrong direction but thinking from a non-existent world of fantasy. Right thinking proceeds from an understanding of the *nature* of both the etheric and physical worlds and is always relative, never absolute or static. Even the coming down into manifestation of actions from the highest spiritual planes is relative to what is possible and contingent upon the unpredictability of men's wills; even the 'Angels of Light' cannot make exact plans or anticipate specific results. The Yoga pupil's own pattern of growth can be distorted by habits of wrong thinking through expectation, impatience, and inevitable dissatisfaction.

A person may think he is contented and feel that all is essentially 'well' with his life and yet suddenly become dissatisfied and depressed. He may not have realised his vulnerability unless he is aware of the ground upon which his thinking is actually based. For he can lose the ground of his contentment overnight if it is based upon any forms of wrong thinking.

Even if a person is aware of his own vulnerability and his contentment is based upon some degree of acceptance of himself and his life, there are times when life seems to become stale or he feels dry and empty, and this can lead to restlessness or dissatisfaction. Everyone experiences this state at times. Everyone who inhabits a physical body comes to a time when the vision of spiritual reality grows dim and the physical mind seeks distraction. This is a time for great awareness and care. These intimations of discontent or dissatisfaction belong naturally to the physical life, and if a person can see and accept them as such, they are more amenable to the reason of that person's own understanding.

Whatever the cause of dissatisfaction, whether it lies in the nature of physical life or in the person's own wrong thinking, it must be taken seriously before it gains hold of the mind, insinuating itself into every aspect of the person's life and infecting other people. If the cause lies in the nature of physical life, and not in some form of wrong thinking, the dissatisfaction can usually be overcome by physical effort, sometimes in the form of starting something *new*; a new activity, a new thought, a new approach to an old activity, or a new sensual awareness of the physical world by looking or listening or smelling or touching, with childlike simplicity. Through the making of some kind of physical effort, a person's physical being can often be drawn back into harmonious relationship with his inner being.

Discontents of this kind, although natural to human life on earth, are not the only or most serious forms of dissatisfaction. They are sometimes expressions of a latent or half-hidden state of deep dissatisfaction in the person of which he is only at times aware. This state may be fundamental to the person's being or even an integral part of it, having been brought with him into his physical life on earth. If this is so, it will affect in some degree every aspect of his relationship to himself and his relationships with other people. Nothing in life can ever satisfy someone who is imbued with this kind of deep discontent so long as he remains in ignorance of the spiritual laws and purpose out of which his own physical life – and all physical life – was created.

4. *The fourth Yama concerns* Balance and Immoderation

This *yama* has to do with discovering the kind of *balance* or *imbalance* which exists in a person's life between his activity and his passivity, and between his various forms of expression.

Immoderation is part of the structure of complex, highly-industrialised societies and is expressed in every aspect of human life, often through over-specialisation in work or profession. The sportsman is immoderate in his over-emphasis on physical activity. The administrator and technocrat may have no relationship to manual work and little contact with the rhythms that obtain in the world of nature. Even the artist or musician may be living an unbalanced life in sole concentration on his art.

A more essential form of imbalance can exist between the different aspects of a person's being, referred to as *chakras* or centres in the Yoga teaching, and their expression. A similar kind of imbalance can exist in the way in which a person uses the different aspects of his mind, where the formatory or word-mind tends to predominate over the child or intuitive minds.

The most serious form of imbalance, which is characteristic of men in western societies, exists as an over-emphasis on activity and striving. A person who grows up in these societies finds that the pattern of attitude and expectation inclines him to focus his attention and energy on outward striving and action rather than on states of passivity or receptiveness. It is usually only through some form of *failure*, at a later stage in his life, that he may begin to recognise the *shape* of this imbalance and seek to redress it.

The Yoga pupil who is studying this *yama* needs to become aware of the extent to which his or her own life is *essentially* in a state of imbalance with regard to this relationship between his inner and outer life. Before any real growth can take place on the spiritual plane, he must become aware of the efforts – and *kind* of effort – needed to redress this imbalance and allow the non-literal, passive, innately receptive side of his being to express and – eventually – to grow.

This *yama* assumes particular importance at the time in a person's life when he or she is at the beginning of the spiritual journey, when awareness of this spiritual journey as such is commencing, and when the balance between activity and receptivity has been tentatively re-formed. At such a time, when the person is withdrawing from certain manifestations of his physically-oriented life in order to give energy and time to the development of new perceptions and awareness, the balance of his life is especially precarious. It is to such times that the admonition to 'watch and pray' applies in particular; for it is at the commencement of new stages in his life that a person needs to be 'watchful' against immoderate desires and especially sensitive to the spiritual protection and guidance which are uniquely his own.

5. *The fifth and last Yama concerns* Right Effort and Wrong Effort

This *yama* is essentially about learning to distinguish *right effort* from *wrong effort* according to the motive or aim of the person. It is sometimes concentrated on awareness of *greed* as a particular manifestation of wrong effort. Greed epitomises wrong effort, for it is any effort that goes into seeking to acquire something merely as a possession without the desire to use it or to enjoy it. Greed is the desire *to have* and may attach itself to anything.

A person may have greed about any form of material possession, whether it is paintings or furniture or antique cars. (But, equally, the relationship to the object can be functional, or it can give sensual or aesthetic pleasure.) A person may acquire books or even knowledge from greed when he is motivated solely by the desire for possession or the feeling of power which possession gives him. People can seek to acquire power or 'powers', or even to acquire qualities of being or spiritual qualities, from a kind of greed. Wherever the aim is to possess, the efforts which go into the acquisition of such possessions are wrong efforts. A person may even have greed for experience and seek experiences without discrimination or judgment.

Greed is the particular form of wrong effort being made by people in the latter half of the twentieth century; it is partly a manifestation that accompanies the breakdown of social and cultural cohesion, for greed is a reaction to personal insecurity and confusion. But *whatever* the person seeks to acquire as his own form of security, it is the efforts made to acquire it that are wrong, not the thing in itself. And the efforts are wrong because the aim is to insulate or isolate the person from the very conditions of his own life which make his spiritual growth possible.

There are different kinds and levels of 'right' effort. Right effort for everyone consists, first of all, in efforts made to acquire what is necessary or useful in a person's life. This includes also what the person needs to nourish him aesthetically, mentally, spiritually. The second kind of right effort goes beyond what is necessary or useful for the individual and may consist in efforts on behalf of another person, or it may be psychological effort made in order to overcome some personal weakness. The third kind of right effort is effort made in response to inner direction, which effort far surpasses in intensity and quality every other kind of effort. This is the highest kind of effort possible for man and it produces real change of being. It is this kind of effort which the Yoga pupil can begin to make during his study of the *yamas*, as he attempts to apply all he learns to his own being and life.

II

Having begun to distinguish 'right' judging from 'wrong' judging, 'right' action from 'wrong' action, 'right' thinking from 'wrong' thinking, 'right' balance from imbalance or immoderation, and 'right' effort from 'wrong' effort, the student of Yoga begins to find that he has a little control over the activities of both his mind and body; he begins to have a certain amount of choice. As his discernment deepens and his choices become clearer, so new desires begin to awaken in him which, in time, become principles around which a new conception of life – in fact, a new life – grows. These desires may always have existed in him in some form – if only in embryo; at a certain point they begin to clarify and come into focus as expressions of his etheric being. They become increasingly significant to him as a new structure in and through which he wishes his life to be lived. These expressions of a person's etheric being constitute the *niyamas*: Purity of Mind and Body, Sensitivity, Devotion to a Higher Being, Contentment, and Study.

The *niyamas* form the interior structure for the growth of a 'new man' or a 'new woman'. They comprise all the efforts that a person makes, from his own *innermost* desire, in order to grow spiritually, and it is within this structure that his new being takes shape and is formed. *Niyama* is, literally, a double negative meaning 'not-commandment'. In the original Sanskrit it meant essentially 'free expression from a person's innermost discernment'; it is a formulation of how a person, at the deepest level of his being, wishes his life to be lived.

1. *The first Niyama concerns the desire for* Purity of Mind and Body

This first *niyama* is fundamentally the expression of a desire to cleanse the body and mind of all impurities – of everything that could distort or corrupt – and to cast out anything which is superfluous and not relevant or necessary to the current stage of growth. Every detail of this *niyama* flows from the basic desire for purity; its manifestations will vary from person to person, and for each person they will alter from time to time, and in accordance with his own pattern of growth. *Purification* or *cleansing* is an *essential* desire which originates in a person's etheric being and, once formed, continues with that person forever. It seeks no particular 'end' or result but is rather a continuing process whereby, stage by stage, what has become useless or superfluous is cast off. Whatever has ceased to nourish or contribute to the growth of his being may be seen, in time, to be irrelevant. As a person's being changes and evolves, so what was once useful is discarded by this process of purification.[4]

One aspect of this *niyama* is the desire for purification of the body in the form of diet and body-care and body-cleansing. In this context, considerable teaching was given in the earliest form of Yoga in the way of principles with regard to the taking of food. These principles were not taught as commandments but rather in the form of knowledge about the body's needs and the kinds of food which would best nourish and maintain it. There were no rigid principles and strict eating habits were never enforced in the early Yoga communities or among followers of this oral Yoga teaching. Knowledge was given in such a way as to enable each person to achieve the understanding of which he was personally capable at a given time, and from which new understanding could grow as his own being developed. No pattern of diet was ever imposed from *without*, either literally within Yoga communities or in the form of specific injunctions. The initiative was always left to the individual person to work out a diet to his own needs at any given time.

The knowledge given to the Yoga student had to do first of all with the reasons for taking in food. These were presented as threefold: *energy* to run the body, the *maintenance* of the body through cell restoration and repair, and the *cleansing* of the body of different kinds of toxins.[5] The general principle relating to these three reasons for taking in food states that everything taken into the body as *food* should serve at least one of these categories. It should be productive of energy or of use either to maintain or cleanse the body. Ideally, all food taken into the body should serve the three functions. Food should never contribute to toxicity in the body.

Four guidelines are deducible from this principle regarding the reasons for taking in food and indicate the *kind* of food most suitable for human consumption.

(a) *Whole food is preferable to refined food.* The whole food is of far greater use for man than a refined or partial version of it. This may be seen to be true in the case of whole grains, whole fruits, whole vegetables compared, in most cases, with the partial grain or fruit or vegetable. The whole is more than merely the collection of its parts and *as a whole* contains something which usually serves all three purposes: energy, body-maintenance, and body-cleansing.

(b) *Natural food is preferable to any form of preserved food.* No preserved food of any kind is equal to the natural form; natural drying is the only adequate way of preserving food without destroying something valuable or adding toxic matter. Preservatives, which are often chemicals, and even salting and smoking add some toxins to the food.

(c) *Simple food is preferable to complex or concocted food.* This principle has to do mainly with man's mind rather than his body, for it is concerned with teaching him not to focus undue attention upon food. The purpose is a mental re-education on the subject of food, so that it becomes simply what it is: a means of providing for bodily needs. The aim is to break the pattern of food-expectation as a psychological focal point in the pattern of daily life. It should help women to become aware that there is no need to spend long periods of time in food preparation or to experience the tensions that accompany the setting out of complex meals.

(d) *Less is preferable to more.* This refers to both body and mental attitude and has to do with the quantity of food consumed. It is based on the knowledge that the human body is better served with smaller quantities of food: that there is more energy from less food, that body-maintenance is better when it is not over-loaded, and that cleansing can only take place where there is moderation in eating.

The third aspect of the teaching about food states that while food should serve all three aims, each food is predominantly of importance for one purpose: energy, body-maintenance, or body-cleansing. For example, energy derives primarily from natural sugars (in the form of honey or dried fruit and some fresh fruit), fats,[6] and cereals. The conversion of cereals and grains contributes to man's energy, but grain is also important for body-maintenance. (If the whole grain is eaten, the outer part is of use for body-cleansing as well.) Proteins are the particular contributor to body-maintenance.[7] Raw vegetables and fruit are the principal food contributors to body-cleansing, but water is considered by the Yoga teaching to be of primary importance for cleansing the body. Cold water is important because it is oxygenated and oxygen contributes to the proper combustion of toxic matter; no other liquid is a substitute for water. Four pints of water daily are considered to be the minimum amount necessary for adequate body-cleansing. It should be consumed on waking, between meals, and before sleeping; but it should not be drunk with meals.

The earliest students of Yoga were not necessarily vegetarian. The principle upon which meat-eating was based is that only those species were created to be eaten by man which do not individuate in separate etheric bodies.[8] This includes all fish and most fowls or birds. Some students of this earliest teaching of Yoga were none-the-less eaters of red meat, for there was no direct prohibition on meat-eating. The observance depended upon the individual person recognising the principle involved and having a need in himself to follow this principle, because he had reached the stage in his own spiritual evolution to which such understanding belonged. Before a person reaches this stage of understanding, abstinence from meat-eating serves no useful purpose.

Alcohol was drunk on special occasions in small quantity, but people were otherwise not encouraged to drink. It was never prohibited by the oral Yoga teaching.

Purification and *cleansing* are concerned with the mind as well as the body. The original Yoga taught that man must learn to become aware of what goes into the mind in the same way he is aware of what he takes into his body, and that he has to learn to discriminate or select what he looks at, listens to, and absorbs with his other senses. The student was never taught specifically *what* to take into his mind. The principle was that selectivity with regard to mental 'good' is as important as the discrimination a person exercises over the diet for his body. And the principle upon which this selectivity should be exercised is based on the fact that everything in the universe tends either to nourish or poison the mind of the man who absorbs its impressions. Nothing is neutral in the universe. A person can, through developing his own sensitivity, become aware of this and discriminate accordingly. He can eventually develop a degree of continuing awareness of what he is about to take into his mind and know whether it has the tendency to nourish him or to distort or even destroy his mind. It means also that a person has to become increasingly sensitive to his total environment and not merely let his mind 'drift', semi-consciously. Such sensitivity and awareness are the starting point for all subsequent yoga practices.

Fasting relates to both the mind and the body, but it has nothing to do with purification and cleansing in the Yoga sense, which stem from a spiritual desire for wholeness. The desire for purification is a desire for the mind and body to become increasingly sensitive and responsive instruments, under the control of the individual man or woman. Fasting derives in part from a desire to abstain from something temporarily – not to discard what is seen to be useless. The desire to fast does not usually derive from a person's understanding but from an attitude of mind which is related to *greed*. In a certain sense, fasting is a 'greed' to deprive the mind or body. Abstinence cannot exist without greed, nor greed without abstinence. Together they constitute a form of polarity which is opposite to *purification*. For purification does not lie in the middle between these opposites, but is the alternative to the extremes. It is the only spiritual way or path which leads to both *wholeness* and to what is *holy*.

Fasting never belonged to the oral teaching of Yoga. Food was taken for the three reasons given, and pupils were always taught that spiritual growth is based on normal healthy bodies not on weak, degenerate, or fasted ones. This is not to say that fasts may not be of practical physical use at certain times, especially in societies where over-eating and gluttony are commonplace and this becomes a way of ridding the body of poisons. However, fasting did not originate in such a context, nor was it evolved to perform a practical physiological function. It originated in the earliest organised religious institutions of the fourth millennium B.C. and has been used by every religion in subsequent human history as part of its ritual of self-denigration or to promote 'visions' in its followers. The physiological uses of fasting are of minor importance in this religious context.

The desire for *healing* and *wholeness* of body and mind is part of the desire for cleansing; it is only the whole body or the whole mind which can be cleansed and refined of all that is superfluous to the current stage or aim of the person, whatever that might be. One of the tasks of the earliest form of Yoga teaching was to give the individual person sufficient knowledge to heal himself when either his body or mind was in a state of temporary disorder, and the confidence to be responsible for the care of both. The techniques of *asana* – which will be discussed in more detail later – were devised to increase the person's awareness of his own body-structure and functions, so that he would immediately have knowledge of a tendency to physiological imbalance of any kind. Other 'steps' in the Yoga teaching, such as *pranayama* and *pratyahara*, also had the aim of increasing a man's knowledge of himself and the etheric world in which he lived. Such knowledge enabled him not only to care for his mind as an instrument of perception, but to heal it, strengthen it, and extend the range and quality of its ability to experience.

The Yoga student was taught that for every ailment known to man a herb exists which can effect a cure and restore a state of health. He was taught which part of the herb to use and how to make a simple infusion from the flowers, leaves, stem, bark, or roots.

Detailed knowledge gave people the means by which they could help their bodies to heal themselves.

Specialist medicine grew up in the course of human history in the same way as did specialist religion, encouraged by man's apathy or laziness; it had the same effect of making him dependent upon the arcane practices of a professional body of intermediaries rather than be responsible for himself, whether for the state of his body, the state of his mind, or the state of his spiritual being.

The desire for purification in a person is the root of much that comes later in the practice of Yoga. It provides a focus for the development of a new sense of responsibility for himself which he must express if he is to cleanse and make whole his own body and mind.

2. *The second Niyama concerns what is called* Tapas

Tapas is a proto-Sanskrit word which has often been translated wrongly as 'austerity' or 'mortification' or 'discipline', implying limitation or restriction. The word is a verb which refers to a certain kind of activity of mind that can best be defined as *discriminating*. But even this word, 'discriminating', does not entirely describe what is meant by *tapas*, for it is an activity of mind based upon an inner sensitivity to what is 'higher' or 'lower' in each situation. This point of sensitivity lies within a person's own etheric being and has nothing whatsoever to do with externally derived criteria or judgments. By 'sensitivity' is meant an awareness of the factors, both inner and outer, in an event or experience or relationship which lead 'upwards' into wholeness, consciousness, or growth and those which lead 'downwards' into increased restriction, lesser consciousness, or even darkness. After the person has reached a certain stage, his desire and will are linked with this point of sensitivity – although even before that time it may express as a kind of vague touchstone to which the person sometimes refers. At a certain stage in his spiritual evolution, the desire to use this sensitivity becomes an imperative and the person *needs to discriminate* on the basis of his own sensitivity instead of from external judgments or internalised social values.

The word *tapas* implies also the principles upon which discrimination is based, but these are never *absolute* principles. The principles of discrimination are never commandments, for the act of discriminating can only exist in the NOW, from moment to moment, and in relation to each particular set of circumstances. The point of sensitivity in each person can provide the basis for this activity of discriminating from moment to moment; it is only the formatory mind which seeks a set pattern of behaviour and absolute principles.

It is difficult to appreciate the degree of mental activity implicit in the practice of discrimination and the kind of inner sensitivity necessary, because such activity of mind is seldom met. It is easier for people to live in relation to a firm structure of attitude or a pattern which defines behaviour in terms of explicit categories – or else to drift from one situation to the next, than to remain open and alert to each new situation. It is also difficult in more complex societies to resist the often subtle external pressures they create and have the strength of will – as well as the inner sensitivity – to take in what is useful and positive in each situation and reject what is harmful or useless for the individual's own particular pattern of growth.

Tapas has as little to do with austerity, self-denial, or total-abstinence, as purification and cleansing have to do with fasting. The discrimination of *tapas*, and the sensitivity from which it comes, is freeing and joyous and is the expression of a deep spiritual desire to be aware of and exercise control over everything that could enter into a person's being. Through the principles of *tapas* the Yoga teaching gives every beginner upon the way the knowledge that he is *able* to select what he takes into his being and to reject or deny entrance to anything which would distort or divert him: anything which could needlessly use up or absorb his energies and so waste the time and opportunities which belong to his physical life on earth.

3. *The third Niyama concerns the capacity for* Devotion to a Higher Being

At every stage in the long course of a man's evolution, from the moment when he first enters upon the path (which means, in fact, becoming aware of the possibility of, and his own personal need for, spiritual growth), there is the *capacity for devotion* in himself. This capacity for devotion is part of the etheric being of man; it arises in him after he has passed through the more primitive stages of existence. At every stage, its direction is different and its form of expression varies, but it is always directed towards Someone Who embodies the essence of what a person feels is *Good.* The feeling of devotion is never directed towards an impersonal 'power' but is always the highest form of 'vertical' *personal* relationship of which a person is capable at any given time. The desire to serve is an integral part of this capacity for devotion.

A man can be devoted to God as the expression of the highest Good, Who is a Person and yet not directly accessible on intimate personal scale; the same man may also be devoted to another expression of God whom he would call his 'guardian angel'. This one expresses God's guidance and protection in day-to-day living experience; it is a practical relationship with Good which is intimate and personally challenging in a way that the first relationship to God is not. These two kinds of relationship form the two aspects of this one *niyama*, devotion to a Higher Being. The first expresses an outline of the individual's highest conception of Good; the second relationship expresses the degree to which he is willing to act from this Good and be guided by this Good – not in theory but in daily life, and from moment to moment. The relationship to the guardian angel is an expression of the extent to which the person takes seriously, and practically, his devotion to God.

Such devotion grows through personal experience because it springs from a spiritual *reality* which has developed within the person's own etheric nature, and does not exist through social convention or an inherited faith. Both aspects of the experience of God are an experience of Beauty, Good, Love, Meaning, Protection, and Truth; they constitute an experience in which all that is positive and growing prevails over what is negative or self-diminishing or dark. From experience comes an increase in the knowledge that the ultimate Reality IS GOD, however much things-transient may appear to the contrary; from experience comes also an increase in trust, from which alone the person's capacity for devotion to God can grow.

This is the essential 'ground' in man's being from which he *knows* God to be not only the *ultimate* Reality but has experience daily – can have experience daily – of the existence of that Reality *now* and of its positive working in himself. From this ground in a man's being and from experience he knows that God will always overcome all darkness, drawing everyone and all Creation into the light. It is this ground which grows and, radiating out, transforms the attitudes in his mind and re-structures his relationships with other men, animals, and with nature. Upon this ground are founded the patience and courage necessary for the continuation of his spiritual journey.

4. *The third Niyama concerns the desire for* Contentment

Contentment, like the preceding *niyamas*, is based on a point of reality in the etheric nature of a person. This point of reality is the essential understanding that *who* he is and *where* he is, in an external, physical, or social sense, is in some way a reflection of the spiritual state of his own being. From this understanding comes every desire to use the external form of his life – its conditions or circumstances, and all events which occur on the outer plane – as a means of acquiring self-knowledge and of growing spiritually.

The initial understanding from which contentment eventually grows only begins to form in the etheric being of a person at a certain stage in his evolution, and this may occur during the physical life or at some point in the course of an etheric existence. It only begins to form when the person has moved away from the level of being where life consists solely in acquiring, having, or possessing. When he has exhausted all the possibilities which life offers him at this stage and has begun to move onto the level where life consists in various forms of *self-expression*, then the desire for self-knowledge can begin to form in him. Again after long periods of time, the desire to *accept* himself and his life begins to develop in a person; from that time on he has intimations of the contentment expressed by this *niyama*. As a man continues along the path of his spiritual evolution, the desire for contentment grows in direct relation to the increasing acceptance of what he discovers about himself and the form and circumstances of his life; it grows also out of the more *active* desire to take responsibility for himself and his life.

But this alone is not enough to give contentment. A person may have some knowledge and a certain degree of experience of the reality which underlies various physical manifestations of his life and still not know contentment. There may still be a certain unease and tensions relating to his life and the movement of his life towards its future. For contentment rests not only upon self-knowledge and the experiences connected with it, but, equally, upon the knowledge and experience which derive from the specific spiritual relationship referred to in the preceding *niyama*, devotion to a Higher Being. This is the relationship possible for every person on earth with the spiritual companion who accompanies him throughout the whole of his life and is called by some the 'guardian angel'. It is the experience of guidance and protection, and the experience of never being completely alone, which makes possible a quality of acceptance at the deepest level in a person's being, upon which contentment ultimately rests.

Contentment is ultimately the expression of a person's knowledge that he is spiritually secure or safe.

This *niyama* is the perfect expression of the activity involved in *Karma Yoga*. *Karma Yoga* may be defined as the practice of using the external circumstances of the life for purposes of spiritual growth.

Contentment is an expression of the knowledge that a person is, as he is, because of the stage of spiritual development to which he has attained. He knows it is not due primarily to external material factors, social environment, or psychological traumas. He is where he is psychologically and spiritually because of what he has learned – or failed to learn – before entering into physical life. He is where he is in a social, historical, or material sense because of the nature of his own being. These external circumstances are, at least in part:

(a) A reflection of his spiritual condition or nature (however unformed or rudimentary it may be),

(b) essential to his spiritual development *now*, and

(c) represent a task to be performed. This is a spiritual task in relation to the person's own immediate environment which he alone can perform. This task, however limited, has to do with the spiritualising of some small part of the universe, which that person inhabits, and his relationships in it.

Contentment with the life a man has and with himself never means blind acceptance or passivity to either. It is an underlying attitude which enables the person to find meaning in all he does and gives him a sense of joy in performing the life-tasks, whatever they may be. It never means drifting, living without awareness, allowing his being or his life to move sluggishly or lazily. It implies conscious selectivity and discrimination in his daily life and a continuing awareness of who he is and where he is – and why he is.

5. *The fifth and last Niyama concerns the desire to* study and learn

This *niyama* derives from the desire in man's etheric being for knowledge. Like the other desires of an etheric nature, it is without limitation or end. The desire to receive instruction, to learn about the nature of himself and the universe in which he lives, grows with the growth of the individual person throughout the whole of his spiritual evolution which is, itself, without end. Thus, the desire for knowledge is an eternal desire; it becomes in time the desire for Truth.

Study is the expression of man's desire for knowledge. It means, in the first place, an attitude of mind which may be defined as *active awareness*. It does not mean reading. Active awareness has to do with the directed use of all a person's faculties of *sensing* which give direct knowledge of the world around him. 'Directed use' of the senses means not merely seeing or hearing, but *looking* and *listening*. It is the *niyama* requiring most activity.

The primary aim of study for the student of Yoga at this stage is that of combatting ignorance, which is the greatest stumbling block or obstacle on the spiritual journey of a person. The purpose of study is to increase his knowledge of human life on earth and the laws which govern it through direct personal observation, to develop his understanding by giving attention to the experiences of his own life and the lives of other people, and to develop and extend generally his powers of receptivity and awareness.

Study does *not* mean 'study of the Scriptures' – or of any texts or religious or philosophical writings. In the days when the *niyamas* were first formulated in this oral teaching, there were no written scriptures of any kind; there was no organised religion to direct and circumscribe how men thought. Even in later times, when religious treatises or sets of instruction and belief had been written down, the primary aim of this *niyama* in the oral teaching was to encourage a man to develop his *own* powers of perception, observation, and awareness. Its intent was to enable a man, through that learning process by which he arrives at his own conclusions, to develop personal contact with the source of teaching within himself.

The aim of *study* within the context of the Yoga teaching, apart from the extension of a man's understanding and awareness, is to develop his etheric being and make him independent of outside influences (for example, the social or cultural influences of his time) and confident in the instruction and guidance of his inner teacher. To study scriptures or texts would have the reverse effect of making a man dependent upon an outside authority. It would weaken his ability to make decisions and to act responsibly and with awareness *from himself*; it would fill his mind with other people's conclusions – derived often from theory and not from experience – but do nothing to extend his own powers of perception and observation and his ability, ultimately, to *listen to* the inspiration which alone can guide a man's life in the right direction.

This last *niyama* exemplifies the central core of the oral Yoga teaching which originated in the 'schools' of fourth millennium Sumeria. This is, that the purpose of all instruction and all knowledge is to enable the individual to become knowledgeable, confident in the use of his own faculties, and independent of those influences for darkness and evil which have always sought to limit man's spiritual growth. As well as imparting the knowledge necessary to achieve this aim, and exercises to develop his powers of awareness, the purpose of this teaching is to encourage each individual person to seek within himself – that is, through his particular etheric nature – to make personal contact with his own inner teacher. This is not any abstract 'self' or source of knowledge within himself; the term 'inner' is used to distinguish this teacher from any teacher who exists outside the person physically. 'Inner teacher' refers to the spiritual guardian or so-called 'guardian angel' who is with every individual person from the moment of his physical birth and whose task it is to protect and guide and instruct that person throughout his physical life, as far as he is able and willing to listen. Once he is in touch with his inner teacher or guardian angel a person is truly on the path of his own spiritual growth; once he is in touch with his guardian angel he is also protected from outside influences which seek his conformity with their own ends or which desire to coerce or even destroy him. In this way the primary aim of the Yoga teaching finds fulfilment.

[1]In some forms of yoga teaching the *yamas* are defined as 'abstentions' and became a set of commandments for the pupil to follow. When yoga teachings began to define the first step in yoga as a set of commandments for the pupil to follow, they reversed the only aim for which the teaching had originally been devised, namely, the freeing of man's etheric being from external influences in order to make possible his individual spiritual growth.

[2]In most later forms of yoga teaching this *yama* is expressed as 'abstention from falsehood'. It is as crude an interpretation of this *yama* as the preceding one which, in a number of Yoga teachings, is expressed as 'abstention from violence'.

[3]These conditions are illustrated briefly – although with certain distortions – in the story of the Garden of Eden, where man and woman originally lived in a natural state *without need for protective covering* and walked and talked daily with God. In this natural state their beings unfolded gradually as they expressed their true inner natures and were able to see these natures reflected in the forms in which they expressed them. 'God' gave guidance and direction to their lives, and in this way they grew. This was the life originally intended for man in the *etheric* sphere, long before the physical plane was thought of – or created. Man and woman in the Garden of Eden had no thought for their *appearance*: they were themselves.

The 'Serpent' in the story symbolises those people who had advanced a little way beyond the majority of mankind but whose wills had become distorted through the desire for power. They had discovered that it was possible to use the Creative Force as a source of personal power and that they could perform 'magic'. When they had learned a little magic they sought to impress others with it, insinuating that such magic was in fact a short-cut to human growth which God was withholding from mankind through jealousy. The Serpent said that man did not need to remain in his Garden, growing only slowly in knowledge and power – at a tempo determined by God; he could 'eat' of the magic power and quickly acquire what it would otherwise take him endless periods of time to do.

Seeds of dissatisfaction, desire, and envy were sown in the Garden, and men were persuaded that God – and the Angels of Light – had duped man and kept from him this knowledge by which he could quickly and easily transform himself into a new being: a more powerful being.

But God could see man as he truly was; in this new state men became aware for the first time of their 'nakedness' and sought to create protective covering which would hide this nakedness – the natural state – from the eyes of God. This was the beginning of *false action* from which originated all actions derived from outside the person, from the desire to impress or to cover the natural state of being or to create an imaginary 'self'.

From that time on, there spread throughout the etheric sphere this new influence of the Serpent – a two-fold influence which created in man both the desire to be powerful (to have power over others) and to *pretend* or *falsify* in order to cover his real powerless-ness or nakedness.

It was after this time that the Angels of Light sought to create other conditions into which man could be placed which would enable him to become free of this influence and able to resume his path of spiritual growth. In time, the physical plane of manifestation was created and the physical earth evolved, and men incarnated (at a much later time), one by one, to work on a plane where they could express and see revealed more clearly the nature of their own beings; and where, through the necessity of making *physical* effort, they would learn the need for and acquire the ability to make *spiritual* effort.

[4]Purity does not mean chastity – by definition: 'pure, cut off, separated'. No action in Yoga, mental or physical, is ever designed to separate or cut a person off from himself or from others. Progress is always by way of seeing, awareness, understanding, and acceptance; and change comes naturally as a process of falling away, of transformation, or en-lightenment. *Exclusion*, in whatever form: physical, mental, emotional, or spiritual, is anti-thetical to the Yoga teaching, where *wholeness* is the aim at every stage. At each stage there is a new form of wholeness, or a re-defining of it.

[5]Toxic matter is either produced naturally by the body, or contained in the food as something un-natural to the body, or enters the body from the atmosphere or vibrations of other people.

[6]Pupils were taught that vegetable fats were most digestible, butter next, and the heavier animal fats least digestible of all.

[7]The forms of protein, listed in order of value to man, are dairy products, beans and soya, and meat.

[8]The primary distinction is between mammals and flock-creatures. The principal reason why mammals should not be eaten is that they experience individually man's intention to kill them and this causes real suffering.

CHAPTER TWO

ASANAS

I

The word '*asanas*' meant in proto-Sanskrit the achievement of flexibility in mind and body[1]; the connotation of 'posture' was applied to this word at a much later date, when the old oral teaching of Yoga had been subjected to many interpretations and numerous groups had developed their own sectarian teachings. (In later times *asanas* became the essence of the teaching known as *Hatha Yoga*, a yoga pertaining primarily to the physical being of man. This is the aspect of yogic teaching which is best known to western students in the twentieth century, and most frequently practised.)

In the ancient oral teaching *asanas*[2] is the starting point of specific Yoga practices whose aim is the achievement of both mental and physical flexibility. Two specific aims are incorporated in these practices; one is the ability to concentrate the mind and direct its awareness to the parts of the body involved in certain exercises, and the other is the achievement of flexibility in the body-structure, resilience of the nervous systems, and health in all the internal organs. In this way the person becomes more sensitive to the state and needs of his body from moment to moment. The detailed and specific exercises provide the means of ascertaining the condition of the body and, in part, of altering and improving it.

Increased sensitivity in a person to his own physical state makes it possible for him to pick up any imbalance, tension, or incipient illness before it becomes set, and the exercises give him the simple means of redressing the imbalance himself without recourse to specialist assistance. A man can be his own doctor. In fact, all the later directions for meditation and contemplation depend upon this stage of development in which a man learns first of all to become responsible, for his own physical being, as far as possible.

The ancient oral teaching of Yoga was first received by certain men, through inspiration, about the beginning of the fourth millennium B.C. (i.e., about 3,800 B.C.). It spread rapidly East and West and South, establishing centres of teaching in many places which then preserved a continuity of oral teaching over thousands of years, passing on the body of knowledge and the practices – with alterations or additions according to the time or needs of different people, but without *distortion* – from teacher to pupil. All this time it remained an oral teaching and was never recorded as a *whole* until the present[3] because there was no need for it and the risk of distortion and misinterpretation was considerable, from the very fact of recording and exposing it to man's formatory mind and reasoning faculties. The risks have not abated but the need has greatly increased for all men to learn from this teaching who are capable of doing so, because of the dangers threatening the very existence of the earth.

Very soon in some places – much later in others (e.g. in England) – the oral teaching was superceded by sectarian beliefs and rituals and a priesthood grew up which adapted the oral teaching to accord with its own authority-structure.[4] The aim of the original teaching was the development of the *whole* man up to the point where he could take responsibility for his own being, but the aim of every priesthood's teaching was to make men dependent upon itself. The institution of priesthood, once created, contained built-in mechanisms for its own preservation.

When this new element, the priesthood, entered into human history, so the actual meanings of words were altered and became set in a much more narrow framework of interpretation. Thus the word, *asanas*, was changed from its original meaning[5] (which implied, and re-called to the student's mind, a series of activities as well as an attitude of awareness in his physical life) to the specific and limited meaning of 'posture'. This word 'posture' – now written *asana* – came to mean in the days of the early Hindu priesthood a particular, seated position and place in which a student could meditate for hours on end.[6]

Looked at in terms of social context, the two meanings of the word *asanas* imply two very different kinds of social structure and culture.

The original meaning of the word implied a high degree of social flexibility, for the student of *asanas* could be engaged in any kind of life pursuit; he could be married or single, of either sex (at least in theory), and of any cultural origin. If this was possible for a student of the ancient teaching of Yoga, so it implied an unusually 'open' society within whose framework such a teaching could find acceptance.[7] From the student's point of view, the aim of mental awareness and physical flexibility – the ultimate aim of achieving personal responsibility for his physical and mental state – was adaptable to any set of life conditions or circumstances. The more varied the activities of the person's life, the more agile could become his mind and the more adaptable his body.

The later connotation of 'posture', which was the Hindu priesthood's interpretation of the word *asanas*, implied a much narrower and more restricted set of social conditions and a more 'closed' society. It was based on a practice or ritual which took people *out of* ordinary life, rather than one to be performed in the midst of all or any circumstances; for it meant that people performing this exercise were capable of devoting long hours to meditation while seated in one place and in one position. By definition, then, it could be performed only by a specialised or professional group of people who, for a time or in part, relinquished an ordinary existence; by people who kept themselves apart from the usual expressions of social life in order to strive for their own spiritual growth; by people who pursued their aim of meditation and its ritual observances through a process of *limiting* their minds, as well as their bodies, rather than expanding them and increasing their sensitivity and state of awareness. Finally, this meaning of the word *asanas* implied a strict and authoritarian teacher-pupil relationship and a ritualised framework of existence upon which the discipline for such rigorous meditation and other practices depended.

It is useful to recognise two characteristics which all priesthood institutions, and all groups formed for the teaching of 'hidden knowledge' and techniques for self-development, have in common. They are both exclusive and authoritarian in structure. Many claim to be the 'true teaching'[8] and hold that the head of their particular

School, Lamasery, or Church is the direct descendent or inheritor of the true Source from which the particular teaching sprang. The many esoteric groupings, which have flourished in the West since the latter part of the nineteenth century, have also claimed to be the exclusive repositories of 'true knowledge', their 'way' the only way, and their members the ones who alone can claim to be on the path to higher levels of consciousness.

The old Yoga teaching was, by its nature, inclusive rather than exclusive; its aim was non-authoritarian in every respect, for coerciveness of any kind, whether through the power of reason or emotion or tradition, would have been a contradiction in terms. The essence of this teaching was contained in the knowledge that God is in every man; because of this, a person has only to learn to listen within – to become aware of, and finally at-one with, his own 'God' – in order to find all the direction he needs for his life on earth. The teacher became the guide and not an authority figure. The teaching was – and is – open to everyone, and everyone following that teaching knew that, in the course of time (sometimes vast periods of time), every man would recognise some form of its truth as applicable to himself and would begin the journey to his own at-onement with God.

II

Certain physical exercises were given to pupils in the ancient oral teaching of Yoga for the purpose of self-knowledge. By performing the exercises a person gained knowledge about his own body structure and its systems and was able to observe his condition or state of health from day to day. The exercises also involved a directed use of the mind as well as the body, for all physical results come about only in relation to a person's use of his mind.

If the exercises are performed mechanically, while the mind of the person is pre-occupied, they might as well not be done at all. If they are practised with the sole aim of achieving a physical result, some benefits may accrue – but they will not be permanent and will depend upon the continued practice of the exercises. The ultimate physical benefit possible for the person would soon be reached.

Change of mind alone can bring about permanent physical benefits from the practice of the physical exercises – a change of mind from 'sleep', torpor, inactivity, to a state of mental alertness, directed attention, and awareness of the fluctuating conditions of the body.

The physical exercises given to the earliest pupils of Yoga were few in number, but some of them were quite complex. No mental exercises were associated with the physical ones other than the general aim of developing alertness of mind and directing the attention in each exercise to the condition of the muscles, ligaments, nerve tone, and the general responsiveness of the body. Specific instructions were given to pupils for the way in which the exercises were to be performed.

The exercises are always performed very slowly, the pupil striving for the nearest approximation to each particular posture possible for him at any one time. He then holds each posture in turn and seeks to relax in it. One posture follows another with the feeling of a continuous movement.

Two kinds of rhythm are implicit in the performance of these exercises. The first is concerned with an alternation of *tension* and *relaxation* (as in the simple act of *stretching*. In fact, stretching the body may be thought of as a model or prototype for all the physical exercises connected with *asanas*.) For every posture implies, first of all, concentration of effort, contraction of muscles, and nerve stimulation. This is followed by the relaxation of body and mind within the particular form of posture achieved. The second kind of rhythm inherent in the performance of these exercises has to do with the flow of internal movement by which each posture is achieved. Pupils were originally taught to aim for a sensation of continuous movement, as in the performance of a dance sequence, which they could enter into with a sensation of pleasure.

Four kinds of exercise were given to pupils in this oral teaching of Yoga, having to do with the skeletal structure, the nervous system, the internal organs, and the physical mind, respectively.

1. The majority of exercises have to do with the skeletal structure and the muscular systems of the body. There are fifteen in number.

These were designed by the earliest teachers of Yoga for the purpose of utilizing the principle sets of muscles relating to the spine and the skeletal structure generally, ascertaining the flexibility of the spine, and developing an initial awareness of the centres – or *chakras* – in a person.[9] These are the original fifteen exercises:

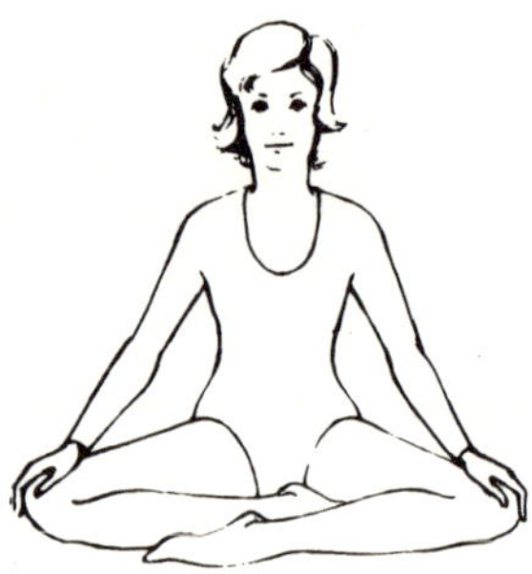

(a) *Sukhasana*. This is called the 'easy pose', for it is a simple cross-legged position. No 'Lotus Positions' or other forms of seated posture were taught originally. The *sukhasana* alone was taught as the easiest and most natural of positions in which to sit for the performing of certain exercises or while listening to lectures. More complex postures were unnecessary in relation to the aims of the ancient oral teaching. (They reflect another way of thinking and another tradition of religious practices.)

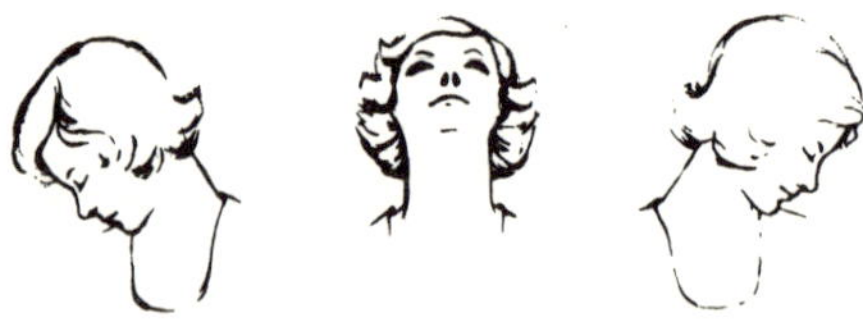

(b) *Neck exercises*. These exercises consist in a form of 'head roll' and in certain eye-focussing and eye-moving exercises for the purpose of enabling the person to become aware of tensions in the nerve centre at the top of his spine and in the contraction of muscles or nerve-tension in his eyes. The pupil was taught the importance of consciously relaxing during the practice of these exercises.

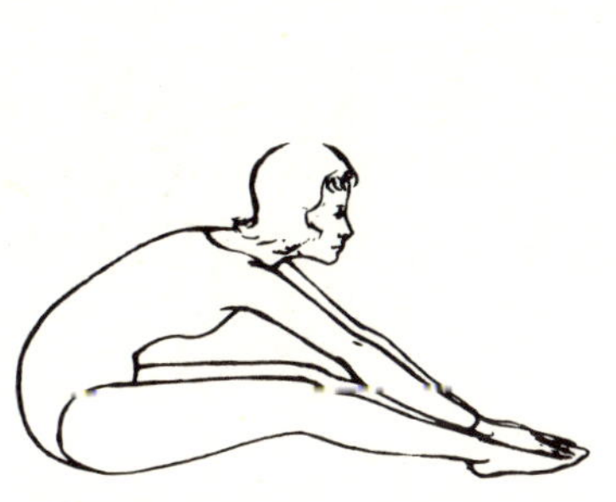

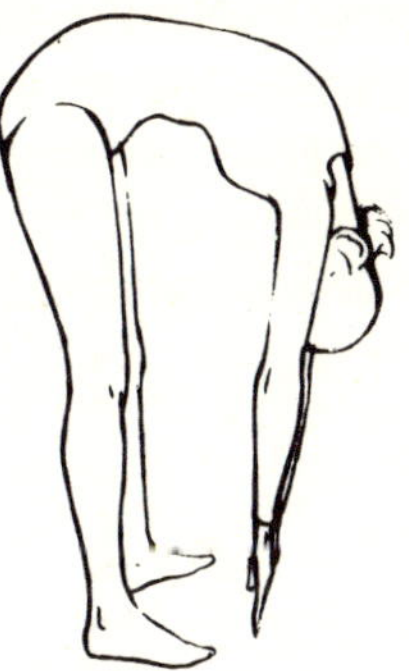

(c) *Paschimotasana* and *Mahamudra*. (d) *Padahastasana*.

These exercises are concerned with different forms of back-stretching and enable the pupil to observe and rectify tensions or rigidity in the spinal structure.

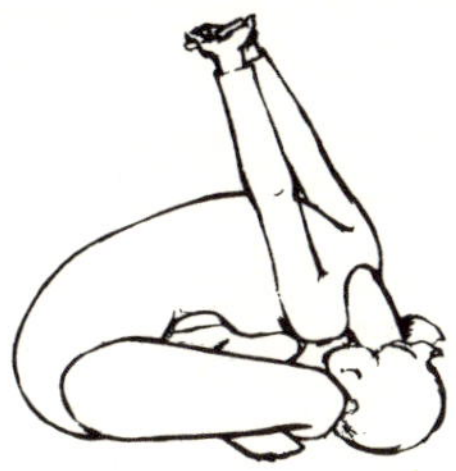

(e) *Yoga Mudra*. This exercise is one of the most important exercises given to pupils in the ancient form of Yoga, for during its performance the pupil can learn to observe many aspects of the state of his physical being. Also, during its slow execution and long-held 'posture', body and mind are brought into a state of harmony and repose.

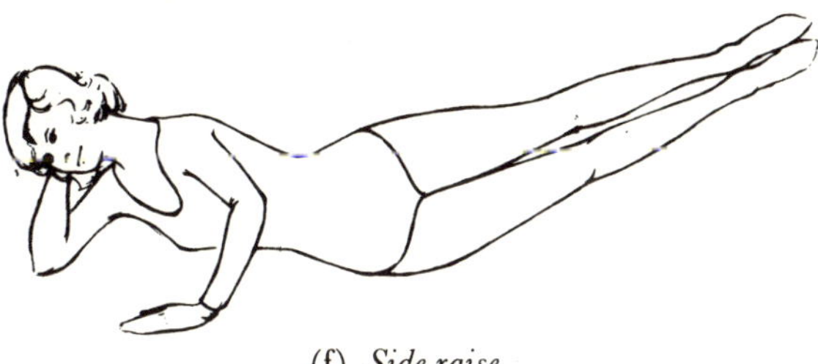

(f) *Side raise*.

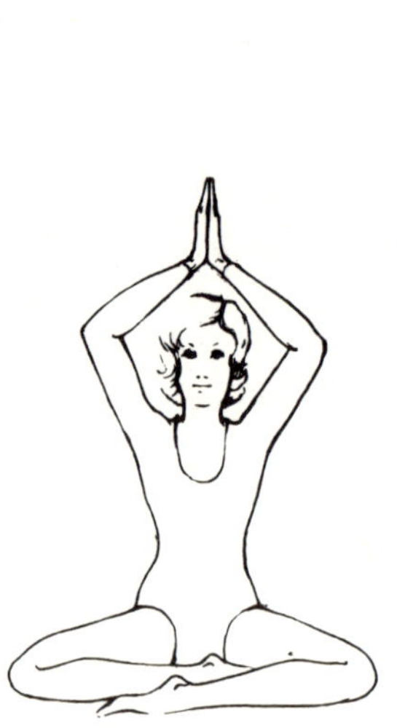

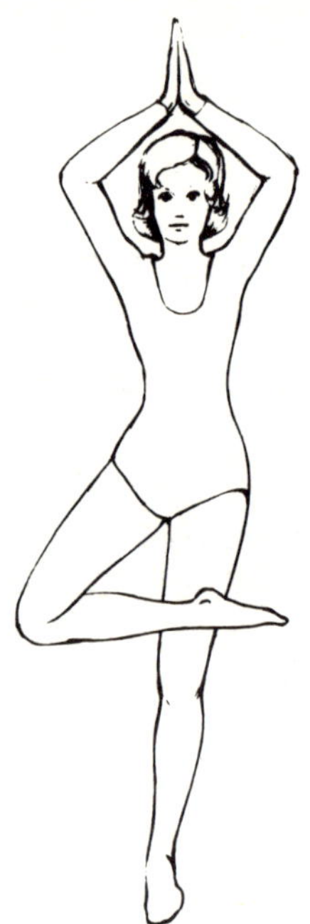

(g) *Parbatangasana* (the Mountain). (h) *Vrikshasana* (the Tree).

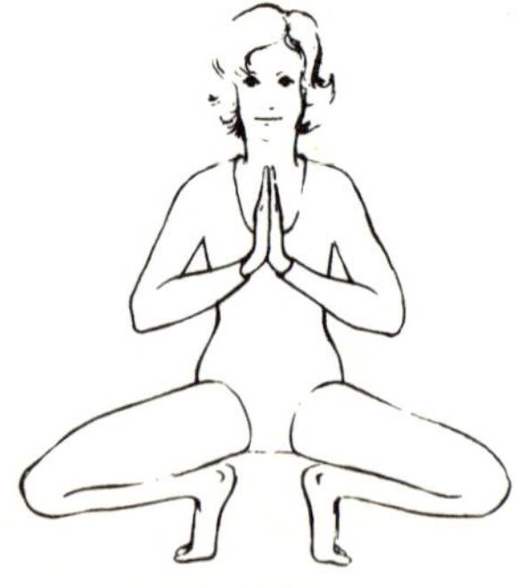

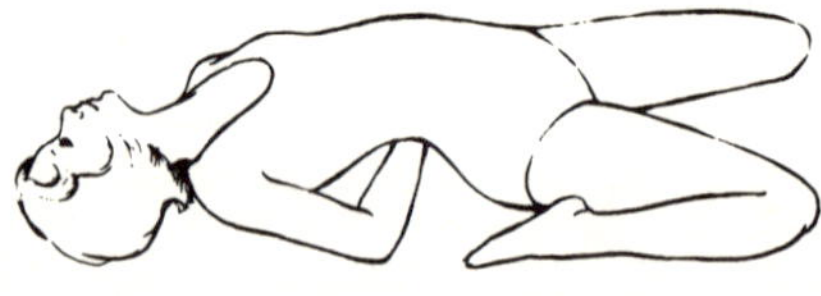

(i) *Overhead squat.*

(j) *Vajrasana* (the Thunderbolt and other reclining postures, such as Supine Pelvic, Fish, etc.).

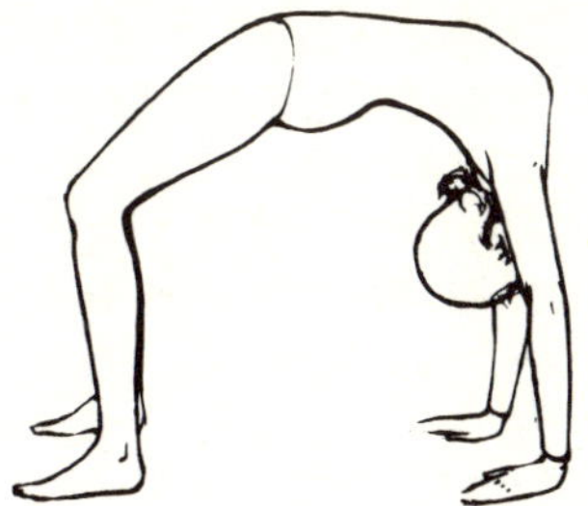

(k) *Chakrasana* (the Wheel).

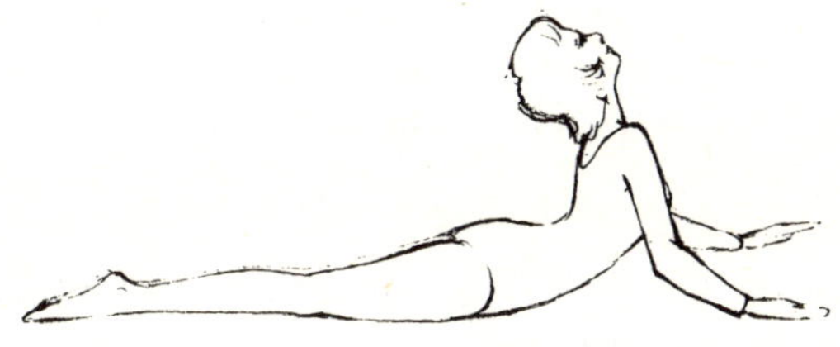

(l) *Bhujangasana* (the Cobra).

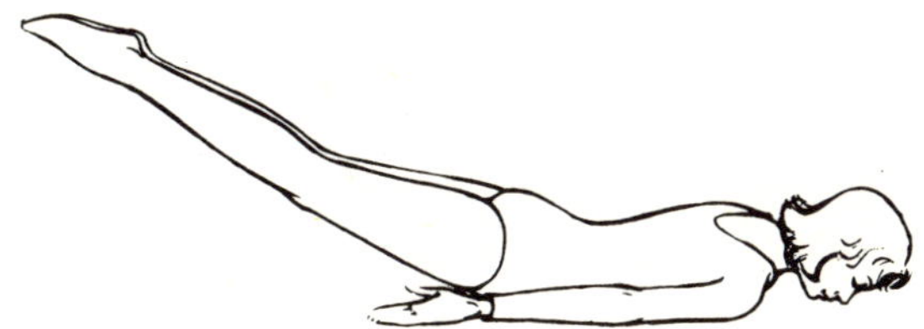

(m) *Salabhasana* (the Locust).

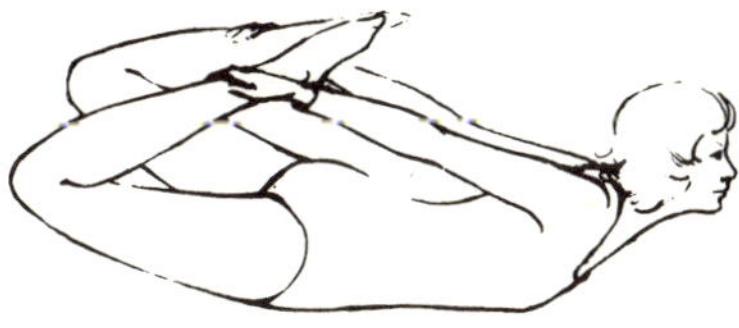

(n) *Dhanurasana* (the Bow).

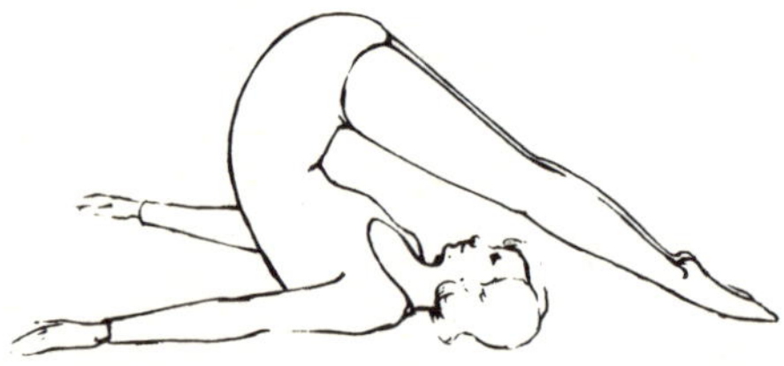

(o) *Halanasana* (the Plough). This last group of four exercises also stretches the spine, as do the earlier exercises, but in more complex ways and enables a person's mind to form a more comprehensive picture of the state of his spinal structure.

2. Two exercises were given to pupils in the earliest form of Yoga which concentrated primarily on his nervous systems. These are *inverted* postures. Their primary purpose, as with the first group of exercises, is for observation of the state of the nervous system. Their secondary function is stimulation of the nerve structure in a person's body.

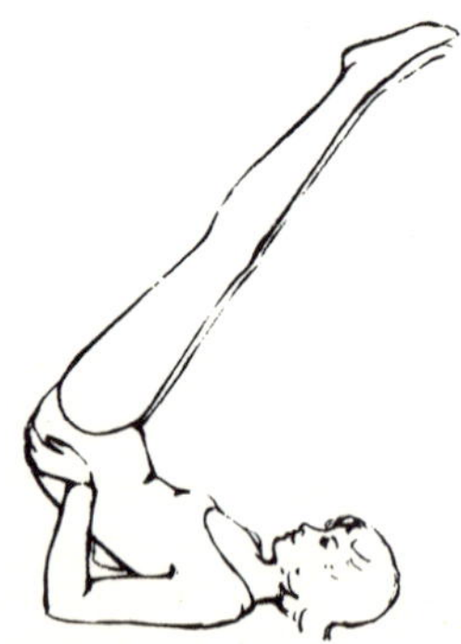

(a) *Sarvangasana*. This exercise includes three different kinds of Shoulder Stand: the half Shoulder Stand, the full Shoulder Stand, and the balancing Shoulder Stand.

(b) *Sirshasana.* The Head Stand is supposed to be practised only by certain people who have special need of it, and not by others. As a general rule it is practised only by students new to the study of Yoga.

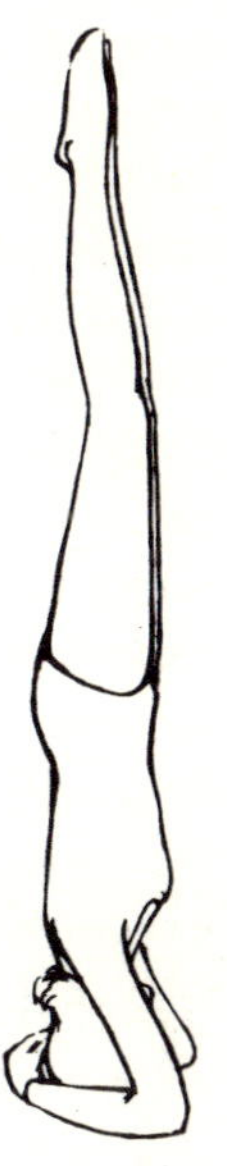

Although these two kinds of exercise were designed specifically for man's nervous systems, *all* the exercises given to the student of Yoga by the ancient teaching were concerned with the structure of nerves in his body, and in the performance of each exercise the mental task lay in perceiving the manifestation and extent of nerve tensions. In time, the pupil should learn to read in depth from the performance of each exercise not only the current state of his body but the history of its tensions and weaknesses. In this way, tensions would gradually lessen and the whole body become stronger; for the perfecting of the physical body depends ultimately upon growth in the person's etheric being and its prior expression through a change of mind (*metanoia*).

3. A third group of exercises was given to students with an emphasis on the internal organs of the body. These exercises were less for the purpose of observation than with the aim of keeping the internal organs in working order. These exercises fall into two groups:

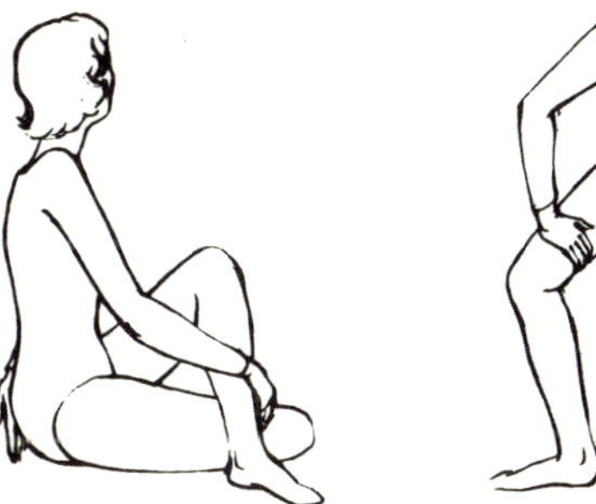

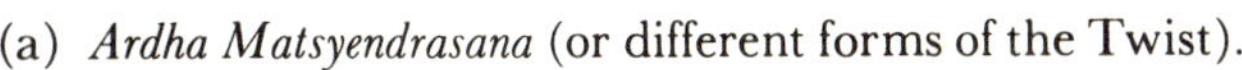

(a) *Ardha Matsyendrasana* (or different forms of the Twist).

(b) *Uddiyana* (Abdominal Contractions) and *Uddiyana Bhanda* (Abdominal Uplift).

4. A fourth type of exercise formed part of the ancient teaching of *asanas*. This consisted of only one mental exercise which is a preparation for later stages – in particular the fifth stage of *Pratyahara*, or the development of the internal senses. The exercise may be called either Trātaka (clearing the vision) or *Shambhavi Mudra* (which is an exercise leading to the direct perception of things as they are, independent of the kind of body or physical mind a person has and through which he perceives life).

The exercise commences with the person sitting in the Simple Pose, relaxing his body, and focussing his attention through *one of the physical senses* on an actual external object (not a mental object). If the person is using his eyes, then in *looking* at this object before him the person gives attention 'without blinking'[10], i.e., without breaking the thread of communication between himself and the object and without letting his physical mind superimpose its own limitations or definitions on the object being observed. What ultimately happens can best be described as an *experience* (the word 'perception' would suggest a barrier between observer and observed) in which the object becomes part of the being of the person in some subtle way (whether the person enters into the object or the object into the person is not relevant) so that he *under*-stands from within himself the nature of that object. This cannot be accomplished, however, if verbalising accompanies the experience – i.e., if the brain of the person is simultaneously attempting to describe or define the experience in words. This is an experience which occurs *beyond words* – or *before* words; *direct perception* is an *a priori* experience which words can only hope to trace but never completely define or explain.

Higher degrees of sensitivity and awareness – or states of consciousness – depend upon the development and use of the *physical* body of man as well as upon the growth of his mind. The body has to be kept healthy and balanced, the spinal column has to be straight and flexible, and the mind has to be aware of the physical state and fluctuating conditions of the body before it can further develop its own powers. No change or growth can take place with the mind either asleep or semi-conscious in relation to the body for which it has primary responsibility.

III

The *chakras* are energy-centres and focal points which exist within the spinal column of man's *invisible physical body*[11] and are reflected onto the spinal column in his physical body; they also function through his endocrine glands. The Sanskrit word *chakra* means 'wheel', and the image of a wheel depicts symbolically, better than words could do, the nature of these centres in each of which a different vibration of energy is created and radiated out. Each *chakra* communicates through man's nervous systems with every part of his body, in the manner symbolised by a wheel.

The three lowest centres on the spine form a triad which governs the physical body of man; the three centres at the top of his spine are those through which his etheric body affects – or can affect – his physical being; the seventh centre lies between the triads and is the centre which links these two aspects of man's nature. The first triad consists of the Centres of Digestion (or intake of foods), Elimination, and Sex.

The Centre of Digestion is a focal and energy point which governs the in-take of all that is necessary for the maintenance of the physical being of a person; it is connected with, and in part works through, the Pancreas and other glands. As man is dependent upon stimuli from his environment for even a most primitive form of existence – far more, for the growth of every part of his being, so this *chakra* is the reception centre for all sense impressions. (Although a person tends to imagine that sense-impressions are received in his brain, they are, in fact, received first of all by this sensitive nerve-centre or *chakra*, which then radiates them out to the physical brain.) This centre receives the three 'foods' of man: the foods of his physical diet, the air he breathes, and all the sense impressions to which he is exposed, taking in all it receives *without selectivity*. (It is the *mind* in each person which *afterwards* selects and discards in accordance with its own built-up structure of attitudes and inclinations.)[12]

The Centre of Elimination is a highly 'intelligent' centre that rejects – or seeks to reject – all that is not useful for the well-being of the physical man. It is concerned primarily with selecting what nourishes or maintains a man's physical being from the food and air he takes into his body. This centre also attempts to reject anything which could affect a man's body adversely or to which he is hypersensitive. This may include various kinds of sense impressions. If he is *not* sensitive to something in his environment, however violent or distorted it might be, this centre is unaffected. In its physical manifestation the operation of this centre is connected with the Adrenals.[13]

The Sex Centre provides the motive power for the other two centres and supplies the meaning or purpose for the physical existence of man. It functions on the physical plane through the Gonads (or sex glands).

Everyone's physical identity, his sense of 'I'-ness, his ego-sense, his feeling of being a distinct and separate individual – as well as the desire to preserve and enhance his different-ness, stem from the Sex Centre.

The word 'sex' has to be understood in its widest connotation. Sex, as in 'sexual urges', is only one manifestation of the activity of this centre in man, although it is its most primitive and aboriginal aspect – as can be seen from its manifestation in animal life. In contemporary man, many other expressions overlie that more primitive sexuality which give the impression of being unrelated to it. At the focal point of this centre is the self will, or the physical will, of a man, which creates, expresses, and even fights for his feeling of identity; it is the driving force of the Sex Centre and from it radiate, as spokes from a wheel, expressions of ambition, power, vanity, lust, greed, etc., as well as the more primitive forms of sexuality.

The will[14] of the Sex Centre – which is the core of man's self will – wills, first of all, to maintain its own separate identity and, secondly, to have its own way in relation to others (that is, to have power over others, in one form or another). The entire life of most human beings flows from this centre and the desire for power.

These three centres, which govern the physical life of man on earth, work partly through a 'centre' which may be called the *physical* or *formatory mind*. This centre is etheric in nature; it has no specific physical manifestation as such but acts through certain parts of the physical brain of man. In this respect it has certain similarities with the *chakras*.[15] The formatory mind consists of tracks laid down on the basic mental potential[16] of a person by all the impressions received by him over his lifetime,[17] some of which remain conscious while others drop down into various levels of subconsciousness, and which influence and select the subsequent reception of impressions and govern the behaviour resulting from them.[18]

The formatory mind of man is connected with *all* activity in which he is engaged throughout his physical life on earth. It is an experience-gathering instrument and the repository of every experience which a man has; it is also the substance out of which the very life of the man is shaped. The formatory mind operates through those aspects of the brain which control, order, regulate, or stimulate all physical activity in a man, namely, the different parts of his mid-brain and hind brain.

All the impressions that form a person's social-cultural and natural-sensual environments are laid down in his physical mind. This includes a wide variety of what would appear to be very different factors until they are all seen as *environments* that impinge on the physical man. Physical noises, sights, smells; voices and words; cultural attitudes, values, behaviour patterns; religious mores: expectations and prohibitions – these and many more constitute the impressions that impinge on and help to form the physical mind of a person. So, also, do the stimuli from the person's own physical being: his appetites, drives, urges, desires, and the various manifestations of his self will agree or conflict or co-exist with the impressions deriving from his external environment.

As conflicting impressions cannot co-exist for long on the same plane of consciousness, so one or the other must drop down onto a level of lesser or sub-consciousness. Also, where impressions conflict – e.g. where an inner desire conflicts with an outer impression – either one or both of them become distorted in relation to the original impressions.

The physical mind is *not* a repository of accurate information; it does not record impressions, either from within or without, in strict truth or as a machine would accurately register the data being fed into it (or receive them without selectivity as does the Digestive Centre). Impressions are taken into the physical mind in accordance with its under-lying tendencies or direction, as it has been formed already, or in relation to a current (even a passing) strong desire of the self will.

A person's behaviour and thoughts are also recorded in the physical mind – but *not accurately*. They are distorted or altered by the self will and by many tendencies that already exist in the physical mind. The true motive behind a person's behaviour cannot be recorded accurately in the physical mind.

All impressions fall, in the first place, on the first *chakra* in a man before they are directed to the front lobal parts of the brain for sorting out, evaluation, etc. These frontal parts of the brain are the physical site of the Creative Imagination in man. But the Creative Imagination in man *as he usually is* (or, as most men are) is controlled and directed by his lower centres and their wills – in particular by the Sex Centre and his self will. This very powerful instrument, the Creative Imagination, is therefore used to select and 'create' the impressions which enter into and build up the physical mind. The imagination, in the hands of the self will, can create many of the impressions and facts which constitute the physical mind; it can create the person's behaviour, thoughts, and motives which are recorded there. So long as the imagination is directed by this self will in a man, from his lower centres, so long will his physical mind contain an inaccurate record of his life – both the impressions which feed his life and the structure of thought and action through which it is expressed, because it has all been altered or distorted by the conscious or unconscious selectivity of the 'self' and other wills.

True memory does, however, exist and all the facts of a person's life are recorded accurately on 'rolls' in another part of his mind, irrespective of the distortion in the more immediately accessible memory of his physical mind. This true record of the person's life is also accessible to him – or becomes so when, and if, he truly desires to learn the truth.

Thus, the mind of man can be seen as a triangle or triad of different functions, reflecting different aspects of his etheric being. The 'mind' most accessible to man is his physical mind, which, in a very immediate sense, constitutes the reality of his physical life. The second mind is the creative mind, most of whose potential lies completely hidden from the understanding of man and whose existence and use are often only obliquely observable. The third mind is the receptive mind, which accurately reflects the facts of a man's past and present existence; it contains the *true* record of his long existence on etheric planes, and from it each man can be guided and inspired throughout the whole of his life on earth – if he so desires. This triangle or triad of 'minds' constitutes the *whole mind* of man which is the epitome of each person's own real being.

The fourth centre or *chakra* in a man is the Solar Plexus. It stands alone, intermediary between the three lower centres and the three higher centres, or between the two expressions of man's life on earth. It manifests in part through the Thymus Gland.

The Solar *chakra* or Plexus has a special role to play. Physiologically, the Solar Plexus is the seat of the sympathetic nervous system – or rather the autonomic nervous systems[19] which control the functioning of all the internal organs in a person and the composition of the blood and its supply to every part of the body.

The Solar Plexus is also the centre of the instinctive emotions in a person: fear, anger, hatred, jealousy, maternal love, grief. These are very different in nature and origin from the self expressions such as desires, hunger for experience, ambitions, etc. that derive from the Sex Centre[20] and are sometimes, wrongly, thought of as self emotions. The instinctive emotions are an integral part of the experience of human life on earth[21] – the *natural* life which human beings were meant to have; they are in no sense distortions of this life or creations of the self will of man.

A person is usually, throughout the whole of his or her life, at the mercy of the instinctive emotions: one emotion abates only to be succeeded by another – and then another, in unending waves of longer or shorter duration. The self wills are internally divisive and, together with the formatory mind, can have no real effect upon these emotions of the Solar Plexus; the will of no other single centre is, on its own, strong enough to control them. If one or more of the wills is strong or masculine in training, and the emotions are denied a natural expression, they do not cease to exist but express internally instead through the nervous systems, usually causing greater or lesser damage to the internal organs.

Although the self wills in a person are unable to regulate or control his instinctive emotions, the Solar Plexus was formed in such a way as to be able to regulate these emotions itself – not completely stop their natural expression, because they are an integral part of man's earth life, but set them limits, help them to diminish, and prevent them from disrupting or destroying the physiological and mental balance in the life of the individual. It can do this, first of all, by acting as a *protection* around the person.

One of the ways in which the Solar Plexus exercises its protection around a person is by indicating what would be *spiritually poisonous* to him. It can do this with ideas, books, pictures, experiences which the person cannot digest or which would over-excite him or be harmful to him in some way, by making the person feel physically ill. Nausea in the Solar Plexus is often a warning for the man to avoid what might harm him.

The protective potential of the Solar Plexus exists because it is a solar centre and receives and radiates vibrations from the physical sun. Among these vibrations is one as yet unknown and unquantified by man; it is the vibration of *peace*. *Peace* is a specific solar substance[22] whose vibration the Solar Plexus is capable of receiving and which can nullify the effects of exaggerated emotion or of any distortion in the person's life and place an atmosphere of protection around him.

If a person is in sunlight for only a short time, some protection and a certain stilling of the emotions may be experienced; but the results are slight and not lasting, for they depend entirely upon being in the presence of physical sunlight. For there to be any lasting effect, a conscious effort has to be made. The person must be aware of his need; then he has to know about the existence of the *peace* substance and the possibility of drawing it into his own Solar Plexus. He has finally to perform the conscious act of drawing it into his

Solar Plexus not once, or only on those occasions when he is under emotional stress, but frequently and even regularly, over a period of time. He has to learn to draw *peace* into his Solar Plexus with the same certainty that he draws air into his lungs, aware of the protection it gives him and the atmosphere of calmness it creates around him, within which his emotions can express naturally but without destructiveness.[23]

The Solar Plexus is also one of the focal points which exist in every person and through which vibrations of the etheric or spirit world can reach him.

Man is an etheric being now. He is not a purely physical being now and an etheric being 'then', when he has completed his physical life. If this were so, how could what is solely physical become transformed into what is not physical but etheric? In order to have an etheric existence later, as he had an etheric existence prior to his entrance into a physical body, man must have a continuous etheric reality and so partake simultaneously, while in his physical life, of both realities, the visible physical and the invisible etheric.

Those who inhabit the etheric spheres exist in relationship to that quality of life which corresponds to their own level of being. They are not separated from the form of etheric life which is manifesting in a physical form, nor from the people who are experiencing life in physical bodies, but dwell in proximity to it and are able to make contact with people through any kind of *personal* connection or similarity of vibration.[24] Those who inhabit this world of spirit and are no longer in physical bodies may seek to contact the person in a physical body for one of two reasons. Either they wish that person well, and seek to help him, or else they wish him 'ill' – directly or indirectly, through seeking to express on him, or through him, for their own satisfaction. The place in the person's physical body through which he receives these vibrations or communications from the etheric depends upon their quality, in other words, the level on which the etheric or spirit being is functioning. If the vibration is of a finer nature, of someone trying to help or guide the person on earth in the direction of his own evolution, it will be received, physically, by a section of the brain (it is possible for him to experience the physical sensation of this in his head). If the vibration is of a lower or coarser nature, indicating that the spirit being exists on one of the lower etheric levels and is at a lower stage in his own evolution, it will be received and felt in the Solar Plexus.

This fact – or these facts – will only be considered upsetting or strange if a person fails to accept the reality of his own spiritual existence now. A man accepts the tensions of human relationship and the conflicting vibrations by which he is daily bombarded as 'natural' ingredients in his life on earth. But equally natural are the vibrations that reach him from the spirit world, whose invisible world he inhabits and who can indicate their presence to him in no other way. By accepting their reality a man can learn to listen to the guidance of the one and seek protection against the intrusions of the other.

The Solar Plexus is a centre where the two 'worlds' meet. It is a vital physiological centre from which the internal functioning of the body is principally controlled; it is the focal point for man's instinctive emotional nature, which is also sensitive to certain vibrations from the spirit world; and, finally, it can become the focus for receiving the special solar vibration of *peace* which can protect a man from the effects of these other vibrations and build a spiritual protection around the whole of his physical being.

The act of being born into a physical body from an etheric existence causes each person's will to become divided into seven 'wills', every will being connected to a particular centre or *chakra*. As long as people are living wholly on *etheric* planes, their wills are single and slowly evolve through different etheric experiences and through many different stages. But in physical life, this will fissiparates and each of the separated 'wills' expresses a different aspect of the person's being. The 'will' in each centre epitomises that centre and creates the energy-substance used by that centre.

This experience of the divided seven-fold will, which is central to each person's earth-existence, was designed to bring about a special growth of will – a leap forward not possible in any other way, or by any other means, except over very long periods of time on etheric planes. The very word *yoga* means 'union', and the essence of the union which it is the purpose of Yoga to bring about is a union of all seven 'wills', so that they work together in harmony for the growth of the whole spiritual man.

The other three centres or *chakras* may be considered together for they constitute the upper triad in a man's being. These centres are focal points through which his *etheric* body functions, and they are comparable to the three lower centres through which the functioning of the physical body is controlled by the *invisible physical body* of a man.

This body is the invisible (to man) counterpart of any material or physical body, whether human or animal or plant. It is identical to the physical organism except that its vibrations are of a different quality, partly denoted by their more rapid oscillation. It is also prior in time, having been created by the creative forces in the etheric body[25] of the person as an *intermediate* body and invisible pattern through which the physical body is formed in physical time. This intermediate body remains connected with the physical body, which alone is visible to most people so long as it has temporal existence.

Some people (clairvoyants) are able to see parts of the invisible physical body of a person (or animal) because its vibrations manifest in colours which define the physical state of that person. A few spiritual healers are capable of reading in these vibrations the history of the person's physical illnesses, as well as being able to observe, reflected in the invisible physical body, every detail of that person's organic mal-functioning.[26]

The invisible physical body does not become a lifeless shadow of the physical body, after the latter's creation, but remains a vibrant ever-moving *real* entity, responsive and responding both to the physical and denser counterpart of itself and to the creative forces which created them and now sustain them throughout their existence. The invisible physical body is essential for both the creation and the maintenance of the physical body for, without it, the physical form could have no existence. The creative forces cannot *directly* create the physical form or organism without first creating the intermediate body, as a stepping down of vibrations from the etheric plane and as a pattern through which to create the denser matter of the physical body. The invisible physical body is also the intermediary through which the physical body can be maintained and healed during its lifetime. Neither its creation nor its maintenance is possible directly, without the intermediary of the invisible physical body. The invisible physical body of a person also reflects all the vibrations of that person's etheric body – the nature or quality of mind and its spiritual level of being, as well as every passing state of the physical body. On and through this body *all* vibrations inter-act and affect the whole person, leading to healing and growth of being or to illness, suffering, and degeneration.

The creative forces (which create both the invisible and the visible physical bodies of man) are etheric in nature and active in all organic life on earth, seeking within each organism to multiply or reproduce it – whether it is plant, animal, or human being. They are active yeast-like 'substances' which are inherent in all cellular life – but not in inorganic matter (which was created by another kind of creative power). These creative forces, which create and maintain all organic life on earth, are characteristic of the *physical* earth plane but of no other planes of existence.

The creative forces are etheric – or spiritual – in nature but are not to be confused with any 'evolutionary' etheric force in the Darwinian sense (which has to do with the growth and mutation of form), nor are they in any way connected with the etheric or spiritual growth of a man – which is 'evolutionary' in another sense altogether. This spiritual evolution of man, which is the journey every individual person eventually undertakes when he begins to assume responsibility for his own life, is *unique to man*: it is not a journey undertaken by any other species. There is no such thing as an automatic and therefore unconscious spiritual evolution for animals, plants, or inorganic matter;[27] no change in the etheric nature of the species is either possible or necessary: they were not created in order to evolve.[28] Spiritual evolution is uniquely individual – that is, pertaining only to individual persons and not to species or any kind of 'group'. It is an evolution of consciousness and belongs only to mankind.

The creative forces belong to the etheric being of the earth and are responsible for the actual creation of all life on the etheric and physical planes connected with the earth. They do not, however, *initiate* creation – that is the function of Will – nor determine its direction. They are not 'a mechanical force that is trying to keep man unconscious and bound to the earth',[29] but a spiritual force which expresses all that is highest and most noble in form. A man's spiritual evolution can never commence from a denial of these forces nor from any idea of going against them[30] – for they are not inimical to his evolution; on the contrary, they work for the wholeness and perfection of every form of life, including the spiritual wholeness towards which men are evolving.

The invisible physical body of a person is created gradually, commencing with the moment of conception, each stage preceding the formation of the corresponding stage in the physical embryo. The same process continues after the birth of a child until maturity is reached. This invisible physical body is susceptible, in its 'embryonic' stage, to influences from the emotional, mental, or physical states of the mother; in its later development it reflects likewise the experiences of the baby, child and youth and these act upon the person's *visible* physical body.

The facts regarding physical death correspond to those of physical birth insofar as the death of the physical body precedes that of the invisible physical body which disintegrates[31] within approximately three days. This invisible physical body of man does not linger on more than three days after the death of his physical body *under any circumstances*. No magic can sustain its existence longer. Nor does the spiritual condition or state of the person who has passed in any way influence the disintegration of his invisible physical body. All the experiences in the life of this person: his thoughts, his actions, his motives – in other words, the total *substance* of his life – which were recorded in accurate detail on that person's etheric body (separately from the distorted picture formed by his physical mind), do not 'die' but remain in the etheric body of the person. At the point of physical death, the etheric body already contains the true substance of his life; it remains only for it to absorb from the invisible physical body the pattern of all the person *believed* his life to be. Nothing is lost from a person's physical life experience; understanding he has gained, as well as unresolved weaknesses, go on with him into his new state of existence.[32]

The three *chakras* that constitute the upper triad are also situated on the spinal column of the invisible physical body as focal or energy points and manifest through their respective glands on the physiological level. The fifth centre is the Heart Centre, the sixth is the Throat Centre, and the seventh is the Head Centre. These three *chakras* constitute the principal way in which a man's etheric body manifests in his physical body.

The *etheric body* of a person is an actual body, composed of etheric matter. In fact, the entire world which man inhabits is composed of etheric matter, in one form or another, the physical manifestation of it being only its 'densification'. The etheric body of a man is formed at the beginning of his creation and does not alter its *essential* structure, although it alters in form and also in capacity (which constitutes a certain *kind* of change in structure and nature) as a result of the experiences man undergoes throughout aeons of 'time' in the etheric spheres. The qualitative changes in this etheric body are a result of the discrete steps a person takes in the course of his own spiritual evolution upwards – and frequently downwards. By the time he approaches the point where an experience of incarnation in a physical body is possible, the man's etheric body will have developed a structure and form which approximate to that of the physical body he will take on.

During the physical lifetime of a person the etheric body remains a sort of 'shadow' beside his physical body. It is not contained within the dimensions of the physical body, nor is it attached to this body by any specific means of a physical or etheric nature, as is the invisible physical body.[33] The etheric body of a person accompanies his physical body wherever it goes, at the same *physical* degree of closeness to it at all times. The etheric body is held in this close proximity through the attraction of the will (or wills) which it no longer possesses in itself but gave to the physical body at the moment when its structure was completed in embryonic form.[34]

The will of the person during his physical lifetime resides in his physical body, and from will alone comes volition. The etheric body therefore has no volition of its own to engage in autonomous movement but is always drawn with the physical body in the latter's movements in space.[35] But even if there is no real *physical* distance between the etheric and physical bodies of a person, and no alteration in their degree of physical closeness, there is a continually changing etheric or *spiritual* 'distance' between them. This distance depends upon the state of the person's will – or wills – and the extent to which this will is immersed in his physical existence from moment to moment. A will which is completely immersed in 'self' and physical existence may entirely forget the etheric body and is not receptive to its influences; the distance which then separates the two is very great indeed. At moments of crisis in the physical life of a person, however, even the most self oriented will is temporarily shocked away from its immersion in physical experience and turns involuntarily to an attunement with its own etheric body. At such moments they are essentially closer and the will – or wills – of the physical man can be impressed with a shadowy recollection of some other kind of experience, for which it may have a temporary longing.

The etheric body of a person contains the spiritual faculties or talents which he expresses, or has latent in him, in his physical life. They are the result of previous experiences on the etheric plane. They are not gifts, *deo ex gratia* – as many believe, but spiritually worked-for faculties (in some cases reflections of a one-sided or distorted development of being) which are or can be expressed in the physical life. They have to be used if the growth of the man's being is to proceed, as it is so tersely expressed in the parable of the talents.[36] This parable, whatever its true origin may be, seeks to explain something about the nature of spiritual growth and the importance to a man of using the full range of his faculties if they are not to atrophy.[37]

The etheric body of man may also be thought of as his spiritual *growing point*. It contains substances which are at a certain stage in their evolution and which can only proceed in this evolution through what the person learns during his physical life's experience. All that a man gains from his physical life, by way of personal understanding and knowledge, goes into his etheric body and is the material for its growth. This is the 'real treasure' he acquires, and it is indestructible.

The etheric body is the body of sensitivity and receptivity. The outer senses of man belong to the invisible physical body, their receptors being transferred to the physical body. Hearing alone, of man's outer senses, has a direct connection with his etheric body. Through the faculty of hearing a person can learn to *listen*, and the ability to listen to what is outside himself can enable him to become receptive to the knowledge and guidance his own etheric body can provide.

From the etheric body also comes the faculty of *communicating* which enables all the other faculties to be put to use. The outer senses reside in and are part of the physical body, but the powers of communication which use this sensory equipment belong to the etheric body of man. During a man's physical lifetime these powers are transferred to the Throat Centre in his invisible physical body and function primarily through his organs of speech.

The three *chakras* which represent the functioning of the etheric body within the invisible physical body are, like the other *chakras*, focal or energy points which are reflected onto the physical spinal column and control the body through the specific endocrine glands connected with them. These are the Heart Centre, the Throat Centre, and the Head Centre.

The Heart Centre is situated behind the heart on the spinal column of the invisible physical body, is reflected onto the same position in a man's physical body, and manifests physically through a gland of internal secretion that is as yet unknown to medical research.

Will resides in each of the centres of a man as a different manifestation of his whole will. The will of the Heart Centre is to create; it is the focus of the creative forces in a man, and all that the man creates is created through this centre.[38] The aim of these forces of creation is to create life – to create the best in all forms of life, and they seek to work on and in other people as well as in all other forms of life.[39] The Heart Centre faces 'outward' for its aim is to create life.[40]

The Heart Centre is therefore the centre of empathy, *understanding* being a bi-product of the person's will to create. It is through this active *going-out* in order to create that a person is able to *under*-stand or get inside the person or other form of life and experience his reality or its nature. This is very different to *thinking about* someone or something. Through this centre a person is able to actually *experience* or 'stand under' the person – or animal or plant form – and know what it is like to be he.[41] But it is never merely a question of 'experiencing' the other person, for the empathy of the Heart Centre always flows from its primary function, which is its will to create life, and the experience always proceeds from that specific vibration of empathy which this centre gives out.[42] There is no empathy or understanding without *giving*. The Heart Centre is therefore not so much about the life of the individual person in himself, or in relation to himself, but is about his responsibility towards all forms of life which exist around him; it is through this centre alone that a man's sense of responsibility for others – for life in general – can commence and grow.

Only at a certain stage in his growth of being is real empathy possible for a person. The Heart Centre is ultimately capable of knowing the *whole* of things and of being a vehicle for the real creation of life. But until that stage is reached, it can be used to create hideousness, distortion, and fantasy-life.

The *chakra* situated on the spinal column of the invisible physical body between the Heart and Head Centres, and reflected onto the same position in the physical body of a man, is known as the Throat Centre. It manifests physiologically through the Thyroid and Parathyroid glands that lie in front of the neck. The 'will' of the Throat Centre is to relate to or communicate with the entire context of life within which a man has his existence.[43] All forms of expression through which a person relates to the world around him derive from the Throat Centre.

The Throat Centre, like the other centres, exists and functions in every human being who has entered upon a physical life on earth in accordance with his own nature. Its forms of expression and relationship reflect each individual person's nature, whatever that may be. The etheric body contains the sum of the person's experience up to the moment of his incarnation on the physical earth, and the talents and faculties which he has acquired during previous experiences are expressed through the Throat Centre.

The Throat Centre is the focal point for every form of communication between a man and the world around him. It is the centre through which all forms of *ex-perience* occur, experience being the *material* of which man's etheric body is composed and developed. The will to relate and communicate[44] exists and expresses in and through the Throat Centre in every person, whatever the level of his being. Sometimes its actual expression is difficult because of other wills in that person. Sometimes this will can atrophy through lack of use for one reason or another, or its expression may be cripped during the lifetime of the person – or even before he comes into a physical life, because of distorted relationships in his previous etheric existence.

The Throat Centre is the centre through which a man gathers all his experience during his physical lifetime. It is through this centre that he gradually experiences his *relatedness* to all forms of life and, through this, acquires in time a new sense of identity.

It is the physical being of a person which, through his self will and formatory mind, expresses the idea of *separateness*, that a man is inherently isolated or alone. It is from the self will in a person that the idea originates that spiritual growth takes place in a condition of aloneness.[45] This idea that a man can grow spiritually in isolation from others has been an integral part of all organised religious teaching for thousands of years. It belongs to the physical being of man: it is a constituent of his self will;[46] but it is encouraged by the ones dwelling in spheres of distortion and darkness.

The Head Centre is situated nearly three inches above the atlas vertebra, on a direct line with the spinal column, and manifests physiologically through the Pineal Gland, about which little is known at present. This *chakra* is the receiving centre for instructions and guidance coming from a man's etheric body, from the accumulated knowledge and understanding which is his own personal 'treasure', acquired through many and varied kinds of experience in the etheric spheres. All inspiration from within or without[47] that leads in the direction of expanding truth and awareness for man is received by this centre and transmitted by it to his physical mind.

The Head *chakra* receives only what is truth – *truth*, that is, for a particular person at a particular moment in time. Guidance through the Head Centre, whether originating within the person's own etheric body, out of his own store of knowledge and experience, or from the spirit world, is right for that person and uncontaminated by influences from his other 'wills' or from the environment in which he lives. For the 'will' of the Head Centre is to receive and impart all that can guide a man on his spiritual journey. Its highest function lies in its potential for the reception of *objective knowledge* from every plane of human existence and all levels of etheric reality. Man is capable, through his Head Centre, of knowing not only what is *true for him* but, ultimately, the true and objective nature of etheric reality. Objective knowledge can be obtained in no other way, except through each individual's Head Centre, so long as he is in a physical body. The possibility of receiving objective knowledge is innate in every person; its actualisation depends upon the individual, the level of his being and the consequent strength of his will to receive knowledge. The source of objective knowledge is spiritual in the highest sense and the spiritual laws which enable the transmission of such knowledge preclude the passing down of any mis-information.[48]

A so-called 'intuitive person' may be someone who is able to hear or receive knowledge and instructions from his own Head Centre, for himself and sometimes for other people. But *everyone* possesses this faculty – if only in latent form, not merely a few people, and everyone *can* develop it to a certain extent during his own lifetime on earth. Usually, however, even with so-called intuitive people, the knowledge becomes distorted or adulterated with other levels of data and impressions when it is transferred for practical application to the physical mind. Confusion exists because most people are not aware of the very different sources from which their mental data derive. And the physical mind, because it is filled with many kinds of fact, half-truth, and fantasy – and is under the domination of the self will, cannot receive purely the knowledge coming from the Head

Centre. This is the state of most people.

For the Head Centre to function correctly (and also the Throat and Heart Centres) there must be consciousness; these centres can only function in a rudimentary way until the individual man or woman has reached a certain level of awareness in himself. The centres which are more immediately concerned with the functioning of a person's physical body – the Centres of Digestion, Elimination, and Sex – can work without his being aware of their working; their wills are active apart from the person's consciousness, and even his self will and physical mind function in varying degrees of half-light and shadow. But if a person is going to receive knowledge from within his own etheric being, which can guide his physical life, he has to become more conscious of his own being and also conscious of the possible levels of knowledge so as to be able to assess and value correctly what he receives through his own Head Centre.

The Head Centre, like the Throat and Heart Centres, develops as a centre only through usage. It is in a state of evolution, and it evolves as the person's etheric being evolves, through many stages of experience. But the knowledge it transmits can never go beyond that person's level of being or the knowledge already acquired by him through experience.[49] Its further development depends upon the man himself and whether or not he becomes more aware of the Head Centre's existence, gives it more attention by listening to it, and, through the *experience* of knowledge and guidance which it transmits, actively seeks its development as a sensitive instrument of instruction.

The three centres that form the upper triad in a man may be compared in certain respects with the three lower centres. The correspondences are not of an *essential* nature nor are they exact in detail but have to do with the way in which the centres function in their respective triads.

The Head Centre, for example, has a certain correspondence with the Centre of Digestion, both of which occupy the uppermost position structurally in their respective triads and have to do with the receiving and giving out of 'food' for man. The Centre of Digestion is responsible for the intake of food substance, air, and sense impressions upon whose nourishment the physical body of man depends and without any of which it would die. The Head Centre is responsible for man's spiritual nourishment – for instructions, knowledge, and inspiration which he needs in order to live spiritually and evolve. But the Head Centre can only function at a level of consciousness not possible – or necessary – for the Centre of Digestion.

The correspondences between the Throat Centre and the Centre of Elimination are less readily discernible. Structurally, they occupy the middle position in their respective triads. The Centre of Elimination is responsible for the maintenance of the structure and health of a man's physical body; it is the centre through which his physical body is healed. The Throat Centre is responsible for maintaining a man's relationship to the entire etheric world in which he lives and has his being, and for the expression of all his individual relationships with this world. If the Throat Centre, for one reason or another, cannot maintain the etheric body's relationship with the surrounding forms of life, the man's health can be seriously impaired and his spiritual life become distorted.

The Heart and Sex Centres are the two possible focal points for a man's feeling of himself. The Sex Centre is the pivot around which a person's sense of identity revolves throughout his long period of experience and growth through the etheric planes. It is only when he has reached the highest stages in his spiritual evolution, namely, when he has entered upon the fifth etheric level, that the Sex Centre can cease to be the sole centre of his identity; at an even later stage his self becomes grounded in an entirely new quality of being, in the Heart Centre.

These are the seven *chakras* of man which form the structure of his functioning as an etheric being on the physical plane of existence. There is an eighth centre – which is not a true *chakra* because it does not of itself possess a 'will' – situated at the vertex of the skull where the parietal bone articulates with the frontal bone. It exists in fact etherically, in the etheric form of a man, and is reflected onto his physical body.[50] This 'centre' is like a door which opens *inwards* onto the etheric being of a person and *outwards* as well, permitting the entrance of vibrations from beings on another level altogether, beyond the etheric sphere. Although little is known about this 'door', it appears to stand at the outermost frontier of man's spiritual evolution through the etheric sphere and represents new and still obscure possibilities for him. It is thought that the door is opened only through the performance of a special act of initiation, but nothing is known for certain. It represents a stage far beyond those stages of human evolution which the specific teachings and practice of Yoga are about.

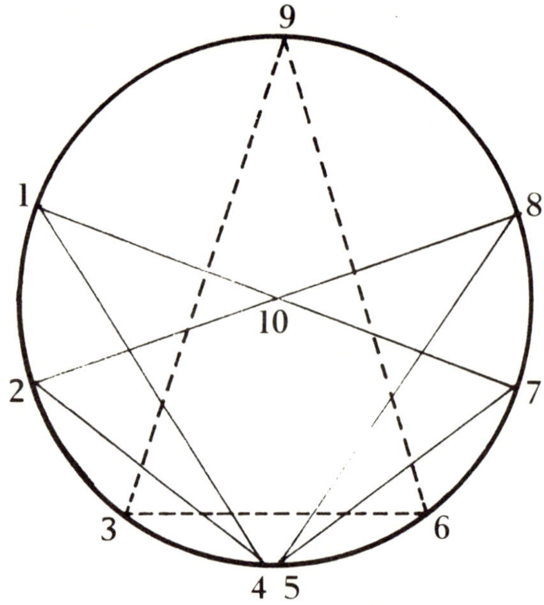

This ancient Diagram of Man's Bodies was constructed for the earliest students of Yoga at the beginning of the fourth millennium B.C. to illustrate the relationship between the three bodies of man during his physical life on earth. In the course of time, the oral teaching abandoned its use of this diagram, when it no longer suited its purpose, and the diagram found its way into other systems and was given new interpretations to accord with those systems. The principal area to which this diagram was carried, and where it was retained and used for several millennia, was the area known generally as Turkistan – in particular, certain centres of religious teaching in the Hindu Kush. These forms of religious teaching did *not* stem from the ancient oral teaching of Yoga, although they adopted the Diagram of Man's Bodies (which they called the 'Enneagram') and incorporated various Yoga ideas into their systems. In the late nineteenth century, a Russian mystic, G.I. Gurdjieff, came across some of these old hidden centres of religious teaching in his travels and picked up some of their ideas which he later built into a system of his own. Among the ideas was the Diagram of Man's Bodies, with the drawing slightly altered and the knowledge forgotten that it was originally designed to convey.

The three bodies of man are represented on the diagram by three separate symbols. The triangle stands for man's *etheric* or *inner* body, the pattern of double triangles represents his *invisible physical body*, and the circle on which both are inscribed represents the *physical* body through which a man functions during his physical life on earth. On the circumference of the circle are inscribed the 'points' at which man's invisible bodies act upon and interpenetrate his physical body. As the Diagram was originally conceived, each of the three symbols represent a different plane of expression and each of the bodies, for which these symbols stand, has a continuous and different kind of movement.

Man's etheric body is represented in this drawing by a triangle which is drawn with broken lines because the etheric body rarely expresses *directly* through the physical being of a man but only indirectly through various centres. The three points on the triangle represent the principal constituents of his etheric being, the creative force, the mind, and the creative substance or *material* out of which every man's etheric body is built up.

The material or substance of which the etheric body of man is constituted, represented by Point 6 on the triangle, is his total learned experience at any given time. This substance is connected with a man's Throat Centre and his formatory mind, for the Throat Centre is the experience-gathering instrument of a man during his physical life on earth and the formatory mind is his learning point –

the mind through which experience can be worked upon or learning can take place. If the formatory mind works correctly in a person it can feed back into his etheric being at Point 6 all that he learns through his physical life experience.

Point 3 on the triangle represents the *etheric mind* of man which is connected with and usually functions through the Head Centre during his physical lifetime. It is the etheric mind of man that can instruct, inspire, and guide him.

There is another way in which the etheric mind of a man can impart knowledge, and there are other qualities of knowledge which are transmitted in a different way, rather than through the Head Centre. On rare occasions knowledge may be diffused through the whole body of a person so that he has a *total experience of knowing directly*. Some so-called 'mystical' experiences occur in this way, where the person has a sudden illuminating experience of etheric reality, of things as they are, or of the inner nature of things. This is the action of the etheric mind, working on the whole physical being of a man and impressing on it a true perception of reality.[51] A similar experience is possible at Point 6, from the substance of which a man's real etheric nature is composed. But here the experience is one of memory or *re-cognition*, where the curtain of physical life appears to be lifted and the person re-experiences the etheric past. 'I have been here before ...' or 'I have met you before ...' are experiences in which the physical being of a person is penetrated by the etheric reality with which he was once familiar but had forgotten. Although this order of experience in its fullest sense is rare in the life of an individual, many people have had some form of illumination in which their etheric past breaks in upon their physical present so that they have intimations not only of 'immortality' but of a plane of reality to which their true nature belongs.[52]

Point 9 represents the etheric forces of creation which exist in each individual person, and whose activity is primarily 'reflected' in the working of the Creative Imagination during man's physical lifetime. In very rare instances, the *direct experience* of actually creating life is possible, being comparable to the direct experiences mentioned above; but the experience of creating life is a totally dynamic one, not merely receptive. And, although some form of 'creation' occurs in all human beings, through use of the Creative Imagination, at every stage in their evolution, the actual creation of *life* occurs rarely and is possible only for very few people.[53]

The triangle as a whole represents, during man's physical life on earth, not only his etheric body but also what he calls his *mind*. Each point on the triangle stands for a different aspect of mind and manifests in four different ways. (1) It functions physically through that section of man's brain specially evolved for the purpose. (2) Each point on the triangle uses a particular energy centre or focal point – or *chakra* – in the invisible physical body and (3), through this, the respective gland 'organ' in man's physical body. (4) Finally, it can have a direct and diffuse influence upon, and function directly through, the whole of a man's body. Thus, the etheric being of every man, in its three separate aspects, can work directly through his brain, directly and indirectly through his invisible physical body, and, on rare occasions, through the whole being at once.

The *invisible physical body* of man is represented by the symbol of two connected double triangles which are formed through the movement of substances from one point to another along a certain path – or according to a certain pattern. These 'points' stand for the *chakras* or focal points of different kinds of energy-substance. Points 1, 2, and 4 represent the Digestive, Elimination, and Sex Centres respectively; Points 5, 7, and 8 stand for the Centres of Heart, Throat, and Head.[54] The seventh centre – Point 10 – or Solar Plexus stands at the centre of the circle, the point of intersection between the two double triangles, for it is the link between the two aspects of man's being, the physical and the etheric. The impulses given out from each centre move only in the direction indicated by the overall pattern of movement, that is, from 1 to 4 to 2 to 8 to 5 to 7 and back to 1.[55]

The circle upon which the double triangles and the single triangle are inscribed – and which represents man's *physical body* – expresses itself through two kinds of movement. The circle as a whole rotates continuously anti-clockwise around the axis of the Solar Plexus (which axis represents the direct penetration of the physical by the etheric world). It also contains a movement of 'electrical' impulses, chemical substances, and energy-matter, all of which travel around its circumference, from one point or centre to the next, regularly but not continuously and also in an anti-clockwise direction.

This diagram depicts the way in which every man's being functions while he is living in a physical body, regardless of his spiritual state or level of being.

[1]There are three letters in this word each of which had a distinct and symbolic meaning in the ancient language – some of which still adheres to the historical languages, such as Hebrew. The letter 's' stood for 'all individual expressions of Mind', e.g., a person's mind, how it is expressed, the forms it takes, etc. The letter 'n' stood for 'all physical bodies or physical forms and their expression'. The letter 'a', which is repeated three times and links the 's' and 'n', stood for the 'beginning or commencement of all creativity, *prana* ... that which is receptive'. See P.F. Case, *The Tarot*. Macoy, N.Y., 1947.

[2]'Asanas' – not 'asana'. It can only be used in the original sense in the plural form, for it means flexibilitie*s* of both mind and body.

[3]Although some aspects of the teaching were incorporated into certain texts and even an outline of it recorded – albeit imperfectly, by the *original* Patanjali (of which the extant writing by this name is a transcription).

[4]The oral teaching continued to exist in hidden places, unchanged by outer events, and its continuity remained unbroken.

[5]Gradually, over a period of time. The meanings of all words were altered by usage insofar as they did not fit into a new system of ideas or a new authority structure.

[6]See the traditional requirements stated in the Bhagavad-Gita for *where* to sit, i.e., the place on which the student sits, which is one meaning of this interpretation of the word, *asana*. Another meaning, i.e., the *manner* in which the person sits, is also well defined in Hindu tradition. See *The Aphorisms of Patanjali*, II, 46, 47, 48.

[7]When society became 'closed', this teaching had to be practised in secret, but it never developed the exclusiveness which is usually characteristic of esoteric cults and belongs to most closed groups or systems of thought.

[8]Buddhist sects are not usually imbued with this kind of exclusive right-ness but give their pupils a wider knowledge of other parallel teachings or traditions as well as the principles held in common by all branches of Buddhist doctrine.

[9]In the spinal column of the *invisible physical body* which are reflected onto each person's physical structure.

[10]Ernest Wood, *Yoga*, Penguin Books Ltd., 1962, p.129.

[11]See p.59.

[12]The *mind* of a person intercepts, selects, or interferes with the transmission of impressions from the *chakra* to the brain.

[13]Only the Cortex of this gland is connected with the Elimination Centre; the Medulla – from which adrenalin is secreted – is not related to it.

[14]Each centre has its own will. The *will* of man, through the act of being born into a physical body, is separated into seven wills. In order to make *one will* again, there must be conscious effort, first of all on the part of the self will, to bring all seven into harmony: Thus the meaning of the word *yoga*, 'to yoke'.

[15]It cannot be defined as a *chakra* in essential respects because it does not have a will of its own.

[16]This basic mental potential is determined by: (a) the reflected experience of the etheric mind of the person from his previous existence and experiences on etheric planes and the general level of his etheric – or true – nature; (b) the inherited physical characteristics from the physical family into which he has been born – which were attracted in part by his own etheric nature; and (c) accidents or illnesses that befall him and affect his brain at birth or in the early and particularly formative years – or are caused by his mother.

[17]The impressions received in the earlier part of the life tend to *form* the mind, whereas the later ones fall on an already-formed structure.

[18]This is not a *homogeneous* centre, and the selection of impressions as well as the resultant behaviour is not consistent but often contradictory.

[19]'Auto' means 'self' or 'by itself' and 'nomos' means 'law' in Greek. 'Autonomic' refers to a system which functions as a 'law unto itself' and under the control of its own will, i.e., the will of this centre. A man is not usually conscious of the functioning of his own internal organs.

[20]Or the *drives*, such as the drive for the preservation or the form (self-preservation, as it is expressed in man; but it also exists throughout all three kingdoms of creation, including the plant); bodily hungers; hunger for personal relationships with the world around the individual man – or animal (for this belongs to the entire animal kingdom and is one of the principal distinctions between it and the plant world) – which creates the receptivity to impressions; the drive to seek shelter or protection. All of these belong to the Centre of Digestion.

[21]Some of them derive from the earliest forms of man's etheric existence and carry on after his physical life on earth.

[22]This substance does not originate from the physical sun but was created by spiritual beings who, having evolved beyond the etheric spheres, inhabit the 'solar' plane of existence.

[23]The *peace* meditation is performed simply by sitting in a quiet place, alone, relaxing the body, and drawing the substance of *peace* into the Solar Plexus on the in-take of breath, in relation to the rhythm of breathing. The mind visualises these vibrations being drawn into the Solar Plexus from every direction, as on the spokes of a wheel to its hub at the centre. On the out-breath, the vibrations are sent out to form what the mind visualises as a circle of protection around the body. This pattern is repeated slowly for a period of five minutes.

[24]The law of communication between people in the spirit world and those inhabiting physical bodies depends upon a *personal* connection in the form of (a) a past relationship while both were in physical bodies, (b) an etheric relationship between the two, or (c) a similarity of vibration which makes them both, even temporarily, on the 'same wave-length'. In this last instance, it may be a positive vibration or a passing negative one which brings two people 'together' – or rather, attracts the one to the other. There may be nothing further to the relationship than this.

[25]*In* the etheric body of the person, not from outside the person. This does not mean that the etheric being of the person actually creates the physical vehicle which he is going to inhabit; but the person *willing* his own incarnation calls into operation the creative forces that reside in him and they begin the work of creation which manifests ultimately in a physical body.

[26]If the spiritual healer does not himself possess this gift of vision, it is not important, because his hands are only the instruments of skilled spirit doctors who work directly on the illness or disability reflected on or existing in the *invisible* physical body, healing it first so that, through it, the physical body can be healed.

[27]Certain philosophers and teachers have taught that all 'life', including inorganic matter, is evolving towards ever higher forms of life and consciousness.

[28]Each species was created perfect in itself, but individual members may be weak or deficient or even degraded in their physical expressions. This is not due to their own 'faults' but to genetic and other weaknesses, all of which are traceable to mankind. Although the species as such do not evolve, the individual members are helped to return to a state of perfection in their etheric beings when their physical lives are ended.

[29] There is an esoteric tradition and 'school' for which this is a central principle: that the Creation which created organic life on earth, of which man is a part, is interested only in the maintenance of this 'film of life' and its role in sustaining the extension of a Ray of Creation – in which organic life plays an important part. As far as man is concerned – so the theory goes – it operates to keep him where he is, for if all men were to evolve spiritually, this film of 'organic life' would no longer be able to fulfil its role on the cosmic scale of creation. For this reason, only a few men can 'escape' their imprisonment in mechanical life – 'for they would not be noticed'.

See P.D. Ouspensky, *In Search of the Miraculous*, Routledge & Kegan Paul, 1951.

[30]Man's spiritual evolution can never begin with denial or working against the forces of creation, as the above-mentioned tradition suggests. It can only commence with *acceptance*, when a man begins to accept himself as he is and the forces which are at work in the whole of life around him. Then can come the desire to become responsible for his own life and to take on the *willing* and direction of these forces for himself.

[31]That is, its constituents are absorbed back into the etheric body of the person.

[32]A man has always had his existence in and through an etheric body from the moment of his own creation in the etheric sphere. This body has not always had the same form and structure but has altered over the long time of the person's existence in accordance with the many kinds of experience he has undergone. That is, the *form* of the etheric body alters through experience but the structure or *nature* of that body alters only as the person evolves spiritually from one state or plane of life to another. The absorption of a man's physical life experience into his etheric body alters the *form* of this body, but only his subsequent 'work' upon this experience and a new leap in understanding can bring about a change in the *nature* of his etheric body – a change in the very ground upon which the person has hitherto stood.

[33]The invisible physical body is attached to the visible physical body by means of energy-vibrations which flow from the invisible to the visible body and are sometimes visible as a kind of vibrant 'cord'.

[34]This moment, when the will is given to the embryonic being and divided into seven wills, is from four to six months after conception, depending upon the stage of the person's evolution. This point marks the true commencement of the person's physical life on earth.

[35]It may lack volition with regard to movement but it does not lack the ability to influence the physical body and will of the person. Because the etheric body has no will, so this 'influence' cannot *compel* or *coerce* but depends solely upon the 'wills' – or will – of the person to desire that influence, to listen, to become receptive. It is the 'wills' of the person which have to change.

[36]Matth. xxv, 14-30.

[37]They cannot be lost altogether, as the Parable wrongly suggests; but this was not wholly understood by the writer of Matthew's Gospel.

[38]In every work of art or manifestation of man's creative impulse is inherent the will to create new forms of life or new life. Every aspect of man's creativity derives from this will to create, although it may not become articulate for him as such. Art forms can also reflect and radiate a 'travesty' of creation.

[39]The forces of creation also work to maintain the life and structure of each person. These forces reside in everyone and are, in fact, the same forces as those that work through the Heart Centre with another purpose. But the individual's body-structure is maintained through the will of the Centre of Elimination.

[40]The aim is not to create *for* someone else. Creation is not the same as *communication*, and the will to create is very different from the will to communicate which resides in another centre.

[41]The degree to which a person is able to do this, without the distorting influence of his other centres, depends of course upon the level of his own being.

[42]Another quality of enjoyment of sensual objects comes through the Heart Centre, after it has begun to evolve, which goes to the *inside* of things. New experiences of texture, colour-harmony, form in sculpture or architecture or pottery, musical structure and the blending of vibrations of sound – as well as of living forms such as flowers or animals – come through the Centre of the Heart. These experiences occur without conscious willing but they depend upon a higher degree of sensitivity or awareness than is necessary to the functioning of the lower centres, through which enjoyment comes – but not of the same quality.

[43]It is important to distinguish clearly between the will to relate or communicate, which belongs to the Throat Centre, and the will to create life, which belongs to the Heart Centre. The first has to do with all forms of individual expression, expressions of different aspects of 'self', and exists to some degree in everyone; the second involves another purpose and aim altogether.

[44]A more rudimentary or primitive form of the *will to relate* exists in the Digestive Centre and belongs to *all* animate life, being the basis upon which the taking in of impressions is founded.

[45]On the etheric plane, it is in the 'lower' regions, where men's lives have become distorted in one form or another, that there is this feeling of intense separation between individuals and between man and all other forms of life. In fact, this sense of separatedness is one of the principal characteristics of spiritual distortion in the etheric sphere.

[46]The ones who shut themselves off completely from other people in the belief that they are furthering their own spiritual evolution – hermits, some yogis, etc. – allow that part of their etheric beings to atrophy through which they relate to the world around them, and they are then at the mercy of their Creative Imagination as it is used by the self will to create fantasy worlds.

[47]By inspiration from 'without' is meant that which comes from the spirit world connected with the individual person – and each person is related to his own world of spirit (in particular, to his own Guardian Angel) – and which seeks to help or guide him along the lines which are *right for him*.

[48]Much mis-information and mis-interpretation of objective knowledge is given in spiritualistic circles and in other ways, through mediums or clairvoyants – some of it unintentionally, some of it because of personal weakness or vanity. All mis-information and distorted truth is received *not* by the Head Centre but by the formatory physical mind of the person which is dominated by the self will. This mind can also be used by the self will of others, including those in spirit.

[49]That is, the Head Centre cannot transmit from *within* beyond the person's own level of being; but it does transmit new knowledge from *without*, from a person's own Guardian Angel and from the Angelic Sphere generally. It is in this way that a person's being has new growth.

[50]Everything spiritual or etheric – every possibility for spiritual expression or growth in a man – is reflected in some way onto his denser, physical bodies.

[51]It is not that a man's physical being is activated to perceive reality as it is, but rather that his physical being is passive and receives the *imprint* of this reality through the activity of the etheric mind. However, this experience rarely occurs.

[52]The only people who are open to this order of experience are ones who are already aware of their own evolving beings and who have experienced, before their incarnation in physical bodies, the unity, harmony, and beauty of the etheric creation. People who had not had this experience of etheric reality previously would have had no memory of it to draw on. 'Revelation' for them might recall primitive states of 'un-order' – or even distortion and nightmares.

[53]This total experience of creating, in which the whole being of a man is involved, is only possible for a person who has already reached the fifth level of etheric reality in his own evolution. There are other experiences of 'creation' possible for man, but they do not involve his whole being. There can be an actual creation of etheric *objects*, but it does not take place in this way. People on the lower levels can create distortions – even monsters – that have objective reality, but the creation takes place through the Creative Imagination directed by the self will. The experience of creating through Point 9 is not one of *coercion* or of *willing* or even of conscious direction by the person himself. For the person's own being is not so much the focal point of creation as the instrument of that force of Caring or Love which inspires the creation. Then the animal is made whole, a person's being is completely renewed, the dry bones come together in a completely new creation.

[54]One of the ways in which the original drawing of the Diagram of Man's Bodies was accidentally distorted by other teachings was to separate points 4 and 5, making all the points around the circumference of the circle equidistant from one another and moving Point 10 from the centre of the circle. Points 4 and 5 must be drawn contiguous – but not overlapping – if they are to express the true function and relationship of the Sex and Heart Centres within man's structure of being. For these two centres form a twin focus for every man's feeling of himself which is in polarity with his Head Centre – a source of guidance, knowledge and inspiration.

[55]The substance which creates the pattern 1-4-2-8-5-7 is a substance which exists only in the invisible physical body of man and keeps it alive. It is comparable to the substance of blood in man's physical body. It was 'created' by the Creative Forces in each individual and drawn from that person's own etheric body. This substance circulates continuously, always at the same speed, and carries in it the emanations from each point or centre. Within three days of the death of the physical body of a person, this substance is drawn back into the etheric body.

CHAPTER THREE

PRANAYAMA

I

The third section in the ancient teaching of Yoga is called *pranayama*. It is concerned with the structure of the created world in which man lives and with the forces and substances which can help or hinder his spiritual progress; it also has to do with teaching each person to control and direct the creative forces which are responsible for the maintenance and healing of his physical being.

Prana is a Sanskrit word for these creative forces or power – the life force – which build all structure on the invisible physical plane first of all, and through it, create and then maintain all physical forms. These are the spiritual forces that are responsible for all Organic Life on earth. The Greek word *pneuma* originally referred to the same creative forces. The Sanskrit word *yama* is concerned with 'commandment' or 'direction', meaning 'to have command over' something or being able to direct it.

This aspect of the teaching, called *pranayama*, concentrates on all that a man needs to know and the kind of effort he has to make in order to command, or direct, the creative forces in himself. He learns to direct the creative forces to wherever they are needed, in himself or in others, to restore or heal physically; he learns to raise their level of operation in himself from the sub-conscious to the conscious, not only through becoming aware of their automatic functioning but, eventually, by gaining control over them *where this serves a useful purpose*.

There are certain esoteric teachings which maintain that a man, in order to grow spiritually, has to work *against* the current of Nature; otherwise, he remains part of and subject to the laws of Organic Life on earth, living a mechanical and therefore semi-conscious existence because the 'power' behind Organic Life *desires to keep him in this state*.

This is a misunderstanding and distortion of the ancient teaching of *pranayama* which states simply that man in order to acquire self-mastery has to gain control over the forces of *prana* operating in himself. This does not mean that the forces of *prana* – the creative forces – are either inefficient in their job of maintaining the physical being of a person or that they are in any way inimical to the growth of his etheric being – or 'desire' to keep him where he is in order to 'serve their own purposes'. Their purpose is solely the creation and maintenance of all organic forms of life which are physical vehicles for varied spiritual expressions of Creativity. Rather than being inimical to spiritual growth, *prana* consists of forces without which the physical body could not be maintained and no spiritual growth could take place at all for a man during his life on earth. Physical wholeness is essential for his spiritual growth.

Pranayama is the practice by which a man learns to become responsible for the totality of his physical life. This does not mean interference with the efficient working of the creative forces, but becoming conscious of their activity and responsible for them in the way a Minister in control of a government department is responsible for all its working – for the overall direction and setting of guidelines or aims – while allowing each specialist or technician to function at his most efficient level with his own specialised knowledge. This image may be applied to the individual's practice of *pranayama*, where a man does not imagine that he can undertake the specialised work of maintaining his own bodily structure and organs but wishes to be 'master in his own house'.

A man may first of all become conscious of the presence of the creative forces or *prana* in himself through his own insufficiency, by way of having some physical disability or illness for which he seeks healing by additional pranic forces. If he practises a simple exercise of 'pranayama', he may have an experience of healing which will mark the beginning of his own real cognizance of the existence of these creative forces and can gradually lead to a more conscious relationship with them.

The simple exercise of pranayama for the healing of a person's physical body is as follows. The person sits in a cross-legged position and focuses attention on his Solar Plexus. He seeks to become aware of the omnipresence of the pranic forces around him and then, on a slow in-take of breath, feels them being indrawn into his Solar Plexus. On the exhaled breath, the person uses his imagination to send *prana* out to all parts of his body – or to those parts in particular need of healing. For this exercise to be effective it must be practised once a day, for five minutes at a time – preferably in the morning on first arising. These forces work directly on the Solar Plexus and, through it, on the whole physical body of a man – or on the specific part in need.

The creative forces or *prana* can and do maintain the human body, as far as they are allowed to do so by man's free will, without any need for the exercise of *pranayama* or for consciousness of their activity on the part of the person concerned. However, when a man begins consciously to direct the pranic forces, two things happen. The *amount* of the available force is increased and something else is added to it through the fact of his raised level of consciousness. This is a spiritual substance which derives from the man's own Creative Imagination and is added to, or enters into the vibration of, the creative forces. Through his conscious act of directing the healing pranic forces, a person uses the powers of his Creative Imagination and in fact sends out much more than what was originally visualised. Many physical weaknesses or illnesses to which a man may be subject can be overcome by the combination of this spiritual substance and the creative forces which the exercise of consciously directing *prana* sends out.

These principles form the basis of all physical healing. All healers, under whatever name they practise,[1] employ this simple exercise of *pranayama* even if they do not do so consciously or are unaware of the true nature of the healing process, the forces involved, and the structure or technique of their deployment. Spiritual healers are sometimes more aware of the etheric forces involved in the process of physical healing than are practitioners whose skills rely on modern scientific methods. But there is much misunderstanding and dangerous imagination among healers who are associated with various systems of healing, with faith healing, or with spiritualism and mediumistic practices. In *all* forms of healing the healer is assisted by persons on etheric planes who bring to their task a wider range of knowledge and techniques than is available to the one who operates on the physical plane.[2] In some cases of highly intuitive healers, and in certain forms of healing, a surgical operation may be entirely directed from the etheric or spiritual plane; in all serious or difficult cases, the long process of healing is always aided by spirit beings. Whatever the source to which healing may be attributed, and whatever healers or people may think about the nature of healing, the process is always the same and is based on the same essentially simple method of *pranayama*. It is the same creative forces and the same spiritual substance which are used to heal.[3]

The first exercise of *pranayama* has to do with directing the creative forces for purposes of healing. The second exercise is one in which a man can bring the substance of *peace* into his physical being.

Substance or *matter* is sometimes thought of as being wholly different in nature from *forces* or *vibrations*; this differentiation is often taken for granted. In fact, however, all substances have rates of vibration and all vibrations have a 'substantial nature' or consistency. The designation 'substance' or 'vibration' therefore depends less on the intrinsic nature of something than on its function, which function may also vary under different circumstances. The function of the creative forces is eminently active, always moving, creating, maintaining, repairing, healing, and so they are referred to as 'forces' rather than 'substances'. The function of *peace* is not to activate but to slow down the rate at which anything vibrates, and so it is referred to as a substance.

Peace is a solar substance that enters into the etheric sphere and works on *all* etheric vibrations – plant and animal as well as human. All levels in the earth's etheric are – or can be – affected by this substance. It is a substance which effects the harmonious natural expression of all life and which makes development of spiritual growth possible for a man that is innate in his being but not previously capable of being actualised. The substance of *peace* can affect the *physical* life of all organisms on earth indirectly, by way of their etheric bodies. It is the state of a man's etheric body upon which the substance of *peace* acts; but where a man exists on or is tuned into the vibrations of the lowest states of 'darkness', *peace* can have only an indirect effect because the atmosphere of negative fantasy surrounding the person – whether he is in a physical body or not – is too dense for direct penetration.

The exercise to bring *peace* into a person's being takes the same form as the exercise of *pranayama* by which a man draws healing force into his Solar Plexus. The person visualises drawing in the substance of *peace* on his rhythm of in-breathing. The *peace* substance has many personal uses. If a person falls under the domination of any one of the instinctive emotions, which are part of his physical life on earth, he can use this exercise to temper the impact of these emotions and lessen their effect on him. It is an exercise which can be performed silently and invisibly on occasions when there is disharmony in the person's surroundings or when another person is suffering from an emotionally over-wrought or hysterical state. The substance of *peace* may be directed to others with the same effectiveness as when it is applied to the person himself. This same exercise can also be used to bring *peace* to disharmonious spirits whose vibrations have been registered on the person's own Solar Plexus or who are seeking to impinge on his life in some way. But it is *not* a method of *protection* for the person against spirit impingement or the disharmonious vibrations of others. It is an exercise to be used for the purpose of slowing down the vibrations of anyone (or of any part of creation) who is in a state of disharmony or distortion, including the person himself.

There is *protection* for man, at every stage in the universe through which he evolves. *Protection* is also an actual spiritual substance which is part of the forces of creation; its functioning, like that of the *peace* substance, depends upon a conscious act on the part of the person who desires it. Protection does not happen automatically at any level, for it is not an *integral* part of the creative process. *Protection* is a more passive substance than the substance of *peace* (nothing can be completely passive or it would be inert) and may be compared with a sensitive membrane or an umbrella, both of which images indicate something of the essential nature of this substance. *Protection* exists everywhere as a spiritual substance, not only on the physical earth. It is a substance that exists at every etheric level, on the levels of distortion and darkness as well as on the levels of spiritual growth – whether or not people call upon its power. It also exists beyond the etheric sphere.

The substance of *protection* acts upon the physical man through his Solar Plexus and can be consciously drawn into the Solar Plexus and directed outwards by the same exercise as the one used in directing the creative forces or the substance of *peace*. (It is performed in exactly the same way, for the same duration, and with the same frequency.) The substance can be directed so as to create a membrane of protection around the person and his own activities or around other people and their activities. It lasts for twenty-four hours on the earth plane, but its time-span is different on other etheric planes of existence.

The protection which this membrane gives is against anything which could harm a person (or animal or plant) physically or spiritually, whether through accident or wilful intent.[4] The exception to its protecting power concerns the will of the person who has performed the exercise and directed its power, for he is not protected if he wilfully seeks to destroy what he has himself helped to create. A person for whom protection has been asked is protected against his own wilfulness, unless there is a *conscious intention* to destroy that protection. This is the only act against which there is no protection.

Prayers for protection, whether offered ritualistically or extemporaneously, have been used by all people, at all times in the history of mankind. They not only belong to men's ritualised social behaviour or organised religion, but they are an integral part of his individual etheric nature. The quality of the protection given in response to ritual prayer is not the same as that which results from the exercise for protection. All verbal or mental prayers for protection, offered by people anywhere – in whatever age or culture or religion, are answered *not* by an actual *substance*, which is part of the forces of creation, but by persons in spirit who carry out their self-appointed tasks to the best of their abilities.

There is one other force that exists within the sphere in which man lives and connects with him through his Solar Plexus. This is the *self-perfecting* or *evolutionary force*. It is a cosmic force which exists within all Organic Life but manifests differently according to the level of existence on which it operates. It expresses differently in individual men and women to the way in which it manifests in animal or plant life. It is not part of the creative forces, nor is it involved in the actual process of creation, but becomes part of every created *physical*[5] form at the time of that form's creation and never ceases to in-form the direction of its life throughout its entire existence. Whereas the work of the creative forces is to create, and then maintain or heal what has been created, the work of the *self-perfecting force* lies in (a) working within each form to create the conditions for the perfection of the species[6] and (b) the development of greater intelligence, sensitivity, and responsiveness as expressions of Will. This latter manifestation is innate in all human beings, where the *self-perfecting force* becomes the *evolutionary force*: for evolution belongs only to man.

As far as the *self-perfecting force* is concerned, all Organic Life divides simply into two categories: *species-oriented life* and *individuated life*. Whatever other differences exist between ducks and roses – and they are many and profound – they are similar in this one respect, that their identities are with their species rather than in their individual manifestations. All[7] Organic Life, apart from mammals, has an identity with their respective species; mammals alone have an individual identity, albeit over widely ranging degrees of individuation. This difference between mammals and all the rest of Organic Life is of the essence and indicates that with the creation of mammalian life some other factor entered in which was not present at the other stages in creation.

In the beginning, the two spiritual forces of creation and self-perfection, were created simultaneously by the Creator as forces to structure and populate the whole etheric sphere. Out of this etheric sphere, in time, a small segment was 'densified' as the physical earth and the solar system.[8] When that time came, and the physical earth was created, these two forces began to work on the surface of the earth within its own time-scale. Their work was by its nature time-structured and progressive, commencing with the creation of the most simple and primitive and growing into increasingly complex forms.[9] This work was *not* evolutionary in nature, for every species was a separate creation.[10]

The work of the *self-perfecting force* was always to strive beyond the current stage, not only for perfection within the existing forms, but beyond them to more perfect and complex forms – ultimately more responsive or sensitive forms. This is the force that, over vast aeons of time, not only perfected the different species of plant and animal life, but created ever more intelligent and responsive structures through which the Spiritual Will could manifest. It was not responsible, however, for the leaps in *being* which distinguished, first of all, the lower animal life from plant life and then – even more important from this point of view – mammalia from all other forms of Organic Life. Mammalian life was the physical manifestation of a different and separate *spiritual creation* to the spiritual creation which had manifested in all earlier animal life. The spiritual creation of man was a separate and *prior* creation to all the others.

All species of Organic Life were created as distinct and separate identities of an etheric nature long after man's creation, and they had existence on etheric planes long before their manifestation physically on earth. The creation of physical form was a different creation altogether and proceeded in the time-scale of the physical earth from simple forms to more complex and responsive forms.[11]

The *first* order of physical creation comprised all plant life; the *second* order of physical creation had to do with all the species of the 'lower', less complex animals. In the *third* order of physical creation, the mammalian, a new possibility of individuation entered into physical life on earth which had *not* existed previously. The two previous orders of creation were created as capable of manifesting in individual forms on the physical plane, as they had done on the etheric planes, as separate expressions of the different species of plant or animal life; their *spiritual identities* were not individual but remained collective and with the respective species on the physical as well as on the etheric plane. At the conclusion of its particular physical manifestation, the creative force within each plant or 'lower' animal returns to its own species. But with the third order of creation the manifestation of separate physical forms of mammal life was accompanied by a simultaneous spiritual or etheric *individuation*, in which each animal received its own separate identity which it would retain throughout its entire subsequent etheric existence (even after the conclusion of its physical life).[12] The *fourth* order of physical creation was the creation of human forms: of those individual forms into which the separate and unique etheric beings could enter for the purpose of certain kinds of experience necessary to themselves and their spiritual evolution.

Every plant and animal *species* and each individual human being had separate spiritual existence on the etheric plane before entering into physical life. But the physical manifestation of each species awaited the perfecting of the appropriate physical structure which was proceeding in the time-scale of the earth. And each species came into manifestation physically as the perfecting process reached its own point of entry with the creation of its particular physical form. Each species began to manifest physically on earth when this process had reached the stage of perfection necessary for it.

With regard to man, the 'time' of his first manifestation on earth was more complex. It not only depended upon that stage being reached when the physical form, within which he was to manifest, had been perfected,[13] but also his attaining to a certain stage in his own individual spiritual evolution before the earth-experience could be of use to him.[14] Until the middle of the nineteenth century few men entered upon physical life on earth before they were spiritually prepared for it and able to make some use of the form of physical expression in which they found themselves (not more than ten thousand people in any one century). Since the middle of the nineteenth century, however, an ever-increasing number of people have entered physical bodies that were not suited to their stage of evolution, or into societies whose conditions were inimical to any real learning experience or growth of being – or entered without adequate spiritual preparation themselves for their once-only life on earth.

Organic life on earth is thus represented by four separate physical creations, from plant life to man. Within the separate creations, the evolutionary (or self-perfecting) force worked and still works for the perfection of form for each species; but there is no evolution between the species. Originally, at the beginning of the separate physical creations, this force sought for ever new and more perfect forms for each species to express through; the impetus of this aspect of the force has slowly diminished over the period of historical time.

As the impetus for the perfecting of form dwindled, so the other aspect of this same force, the evolutionary impulse, has grown in strength. Not that the possibility of evolution between the separate creations ever existed – or ever will do so. It exists only within the separate creation of man and works only within *individual* men and women – not on the species as such – as a force that reinforces each person's own will to grow and evolve spiritually. The evolutionary force has itself evolved; it is a more evolved stage of the self-perfecting force. For 'perfection' in man is not a specialised physical form with a certain kind of intelligence, nor even a particular etheric expression of Life. Perfection for man is individual and unique, a continuous growth of being: of sensitivity, responsiveness, and the will to assume personal responsibility. It is a growth that is without limits or finiteness.

The plant and animal species, and the individuated mammals within their species, are intrinsically *spiritual* creations and beings; as such, they are not subject to the laws governing physical life on earth. As far as they are concerned, the self-perfecting or evolutionary force works solely within the structure of physical life on earth and is subject to its laws, conditions, and time-scale. This force cannot alter the etheric reality of plant or animal life or effect spiritual changes. These species and the individuated animal forms were created spiritually perfect and do not in any way evolve – or need to evolve – from one spiritual form to another, either in their earth experience or on the spiritual plane where their existence continues for eternity in the etheric body of Organic Life as a whole.[15] But the *physical* manifestations of Organic Life are not perfect, as they were intended to be, because of the conditions which men have allowed to develop and the states of greed and violence which man has created. Man's vibrations have distorted the physical manifestations and behaviour of both plant and animal life on earth; because of their sensitivity, plants and animals have picked up or in-breathed these vibrations so that their own physical expressions have become distorted to a point of considerable variance with their spiritual beings.[16] After their lives in physical bodies are completed, all animals or animal species have to be spiritually cleansed of these vibrations and of their un-natural behaviour patterns before being able to continue their normal spiritual existence on the etheric plane.

It is difficult for human beings, whose minds are structured by ideas of change and growth, to accept the existence of life which does not alter in its etheric nature but simply has been *as it is* for all time. It does not fit into his conceptual world. But the fact is that all Organic Life, plant and animal, does not need to 'go anywhere' spiritually nor is it subject to any state of change; and yet it is never static but is always moving in accordance with its own intrinsic nature.

At the same time Organic Life on earth expresses physically, in so many different ways, this concept of growth and evolution. It was created in part for the purpose of so impressing on man an awareness of growth as to awaken his own desire for *spiritual* growth and remind him of his true nature and purpose. All physical life expresses a birth-growth-death-rebirth cycle which is not reflective of the spiritual nature of any species nor of etheric life in general. Organic Life on earth has, in a sense, 'taken on' this task for the benefit of man; for the earth can be seen as his spiritual 'forcing house', where physical experience can sharpen and clarify the choices open to him and create the conditions in which individuals can will their own spiritual growth.

II

The lower centres in a man revolve around, and derive their meaning from, his self will. The self will of a person controls his life from its centre in the Sex *chakra*, incorporating his sense of identity and his desire for power which are integral to it. The self will is always changing form or discovering new interests through which to express; the desire for power finds limitless avenues for expression which can be masked by varied faces of compliancy, consideration, and even self awareness. The self will changes form but is nonetheless always present somewhere, with a grip on the person and his life. Not even the light of consciousness can actually *free* the person from the grip of this will.

Yet there comes a turning point for the student of yoga when some change is possible, when the essential being of a man begins to make itself felt more decisively not only through the higher centres in him but in other ways as well. Up to this point, while the person has tried to understand and practise the *yamas* and *niyamas*, as well as he could, and endeavoured to acquire both flexibility of and control over his mind and body (which work on the *asanas* implies), the self will has been both participant and partial beneficiary. The person has become more aware in his relationships with other people and his attitudes towards them have altered. There have been many changes in his thinking about himself and in the structure of his physical life. There are encouraging signs and proofs that the person is on the right journey – on the right road for himself. And yet, in many different ways, the old will still reveals itself characteristically. So much has changed, and yet the old self is still around.

The turning point comes when the etheric being or nature of the man – all he has brought with him into his physical life from previous experiences and the knowledge he has acquired from long existence on etheric planes – starts to impress itself on his consciousness through his *kundalini sense.* This 'sense' is latent in the Sex Centre of every person. It is a focal point through which the true nature of a person and his own real, although previously hidden knowledge can express.

When the *kundalini sense* begins to function, it manifests internally, within the person himself, and causes him to experience another order of reality which does not readily fit into his physical life pattern; nor is it comprehensible in terms of his ordinary thinking. These experiences, which happen in a person through the *kundalini sense*, can therefore challenge the very authority of the self will on which his physical life is based, because they are reflections of the true nature of his being: they are expressions of his own reality, *whatever the stage of its development.*

The word *kundalini* is found in both ancient and contemporary Yoga literature[17] where it usually refers to a latent energy or power 'curled up like a serpent at the base of the spine'[18] which, when awakened, is supposed to travel up the spine through the *chakras* and give rise to psychic powers and higher states of consciousness. This is, however, a very misleading conception which can encourage dangerous fantasies in people who take it seriously or seek such powers.

The word *kundalini* means, in general, something which is potential or latent. It is not, in fact, an energy or power at all but a kind of 'sense' or sensitive point which exists in man's Sex Centre and picks up vibrations from his etheric being which refer to its real nature and the experiences which had previously gone into its formation. This sense exists in the Sex Centre because it is man's centre of gravity for most of his evolution and there must be a way in which his own true nature and etheric being can get through to him. Thus, through this sense a man may re-experience portions of experiences he has had over aeons of time and which have gone into the making of his being at its present stage. Through this process of re-experiencing he can also become aware of the actual existence of his etheric being and may eventually be able to make a conscious connection with it; he is likewise slowly reminded of the purpose or meaning implicit in his etheric existence, and so the perspective from which he regards his present physical life can begin to alter. In time, this physical life of a man may come to be experienced in relation to the purpose and needs of his etheric being. His physical life can then become more essentially a spiritual journey.

If the experiences belonging to a man's etheric being, and picked up by his *kundalini sense*, are not understood as such they can become distorted by the self will and contribute to its imagination about itself. His sense of self then becomes filled with the energy with which these new revelations are charged[19] and he seems to himself to be filled with power. If the *kundalini sense* is swamped in this way by the man's Sex Centre and everything that feeds and gives identity to his physical self, it is no longer capable of picking up the more subtle vibrations from his inner, etheric being. His life again becomes directed wholly outwards towards the acquisition of power for the self, and the opportunity for re-establishing contact with his real self is past – at least for the time being. Another opportunity for the functioning of his *kundalini sense* may become possible later, but only during some crisis in the course of his physical life.

There can be no alteration in the structure and direction of a man's physical life on earth – and no permanent change in the nature of his real inner being, with which he entered upon that life – except through the *kundalini sense* and the right development of its sensitivity. Many factors in a man's physical life, which do not belong to his inner nature, contribute to the development of his physical self and all that identifies him to himself and others on the physical plane. This self, in which is centred his self will, can only perpetuate itself – never change itself. Even the creative forces in a man, which created and then maintain his physical body, have no power to bring about *spiritual* changes. The nature of an individual as he is, at any particular stage in his evolution as an etheric being, can only change through a change in what he *wills*. And an alteration in the nature of his willing only comes about through an increase in his awareness of himself, which is a result of renewed contact with his true nature in the midst of his physical life. This contact – which comes through his *kundalini sense* – gradually restores to him contact with his own unique knowledge and prior experience which make possible a change in the nature and direction of his willing. It is this change which is the purpose of every man's physical life on earth.

The etheric being of a man manifests *directly* on his physical life in three different ways and through three separate focal points: his Creative Imagination, his Head Centre, and the *kundalini sense*. All three are important for the change in direction which marks the commencement of his evolution and for its continuation. If his etheric being expressed only through his Creative Imagination, the person would have no awareness of the *nature* of his own etheric being and no inner guidance and he would create new images of self, new phantasies, or even monsters! If his etheric being manifested only through the Head Centre, its guidance and perception of reality would be abstract or theoretical because it was not related to the man's own nature, that is, to any experience or awareness of his own true substance. Such abstract 'inspiration' could create a dichotomy in the man's experience of himself, whereby the expressions of his lower centres and his physical life generally would be seen as *opposed to* the information which came through his Head Centre; or else such 'inspiration' would produce no result at all. This is the dualism in which some philosophers and theologians profess to believe but which has no real basis in man's own nature. *Experience* of the nature and state of his own etheric or real being, through the *kundalini sense*, is therefore essential for a man before any real change can take place in the direction of what he wills and in the structure of his self will. After that the perceptions which the increased sensitivity of his Head Centre makes possible fall on his awareness of and knowledge about himself, and his own creative force – his Creative Imagination – can be used to actualise the next stage in his spiritual growth.

The self will of a man cannot be defined solely in terms of his lower centres and the physical expression of his life, although for a long time – and with many people for most of their lives – the self is circumscribed by the lower centres, the Sex Centre in particular. The self will is, in essence, the expression of a man's etheric being – a reflection of his Divine Will or, rather, the form in which it appears during his physical life on earth. There is no other will in a man during his physical life on earth except his self will; it *alone* is the expression of his Divine Will. Even if the direction of its expression is wholly outwards and determined by the man's material life, it is nonetheless a reflection of the inner or etheric nature of that man. There is *no* built-in dualism in a man which consists of two wills, one 'outer' and the other reflecting an inward-facing or spiritual desire. And yet his *willing* is not singular but composed of a multiplicity of desires which, taken together, determine the nature of the will and its direction from moment to moment. For any change to take place in a man's nature, there must first of all be a change in the nature of his willing, which means a consolidation of one group of desires to give consistent direction to his willing.

When the *kundalini sense* is awakened in a person, the knowledge inherent in his own inner being returns to him slowly. It is this knowledge which can, in time, bring about a change in the nature of his self will. It is possible for this process to commence in any person whatever his level of being, but it occurs more frequently in those people in whom an awareness has already begun to develop that their lives are concerned with some kind of spiritual growth. For anyone who, before entering upon a physical life, had begun to evolve perceptions that lead beyond self having or self expression, this is a most important time. When the *kundalini sense* begins to function in the physical life, he can be reminded from then on, in one way or another, of the etheric experiences which led to and inspired his spiritual growth. It is important for the Yoga pupil to become conscious of this process of awakening and recovery in himself and its true nature.

The *kundalini sense* is at work in all people *to a certain degree* from the commencement of their lives. For it to manifest more fully, imparting the experiences and nature of the person's etheric being, there must be awareness on the part of that person. The question for everyone, therefore, at a certain stage, becomes one of identifying the *kundalini sense* in himself, distinguishing the various forms in which it manifests and has manifested throughout his life, and recognising that this is the way in which his own inner being has been endeavouring to reveal itself to him.

There are various indications of its presence. One form in which the *kundalini sense* expresses itself is as a sometimes vague but nonetheless distinctive longing or nostalgia for something 'lost'. This can manifest in different ways, expressing (in Western cultures) pantheistically, religiously, or sexually. (The *forms* of expression are not intrinsic to the *kundalini sense* but rather modes of expression characteristic of these cultures.) The longing for union with nature is largely a spiritual longing or the expression of a person's inner being. The idealised Man or Woman – the image of all that is good, true, perfect, with whom the sexually maturing young person identifies himself – is also largely an expression of the person's inner being.[20] *Religious* expressions of the *kundalini sense* have filled literature with the love imagery of the devotee or mystic from earliest times. The Spiritual Marriage, the longing of the Bride for the

Bridegroom, the Mystical Union with Christ are some of the many descriptions of a person's response to intimations of spiritual reality in himself. Underlying these forms of expression is the unconscious desire for spiritual growth; but this desire may be externalised and draw the man away from perceiving the true nature of his longing onto a plane where satisfaction is short-lived and fulfilment impossible.

One difficulty for the person lies in distinguishing the fact of the *kundalini sense*, and what it is revealing to a man about the nature of his own being, from his fantasies and the cultural or religious forms in which his fantasies are expressed.

Mystical experience describes a form of human experience which is as old as mankind. The term is often used to refer, in particular, to the Mysteries of Greece and Rome, or to the Egyptian Mysteries, and implies a body of hidden or secret or sacred knowledge. These Mysteries were based on a certain body of knowledge or ancient teaching, hidden from most people but passed on from High Priest to High Priest, or from guru to pupil, by way of certain schools of learning and various forms of initiation. All religions have their 'secret' or esoteric aspect and schools for the teaching of a sacred or hidden body of knowledge exist – and have always existed – in most highly-developed cultures. Their existence depends in part upon that innate desire in man for secrecy and the sense of personal power which the possession of secret knowledge gives him.[21] But, even more than that, the perpetuation of all esoteric schools and teachings – all Mysteries – depends upon (1) the need to preserve in its entirety a certain body of knowledge about man and the conditions necessary for his spiritual evolution, (2) the desire of individual persons for self-knowledge, and (3) the desire to acquire special powers or a higher level of consciousness. These esoteric teachings and their rites of initiation, whatever the form of their manifestation, depend upon a correlation of outer and inner: of external form with the interior state of mind of the individual person. But however close the correlation of outer with inner might be, a form could never exist within which the etheric being of an individual could grow or evolve *naturally*, for the requirements of any 'school' of teaching will always impose on him its own conceptual pattern. Even a person who, out of the strongest desire for truth, joined such a school would, on becoming a pupil, lose the possibility of making free contact with his own conscience and his own etheric nature – out of which contact alone can come true spiritual growth.[22]

Such was the teaching of the one called Christ who taught that the direction for a man's new growth and wholeness lay within his own being. His *real* teaching was about the growth of each person's own unique being out of his own knowledge and experience and free from any external form of coercion. The essence of this teaching lay in showing each man how to take personal responsibility for himself and his life.

Another manifestation of the *kundalini sense* lies in certain kinds of dreams which are considered erotic by some schools of modern psychology but are, in some people, intimations of their inner reality and the awakening desire to contact – to feel, to touch – their own inner beings. An idealised form of the opposite sex often appears in these dreams – usually someone unknown to the dreamer, with whom he or she is in complete and intimate harmony. If sexual desire enters into this situation it rarely expresses itself in the sexual act but rather in a passive lying together. In fact, the Stranger in the dream, whether male or female, is always passive and never sexually domineering. The need expressed in such dreams is for *contact*, for harmony or at-onement – never for sexual excitement, even if the latter occasionally takes over and colours the dream.

These dreams occur not only in adolescence or early adulthood, but may continue throughout the whole of a person's life and are very upsetting to someone in the middle years if their origin is not recognised or their purpose understood. For they are not always expressions of biological sexual frustration, where the indicated remedy lies in the direction of new sexual experience or a different partner. The dream may be an expression of the person's own *kundalini sense* and can recall in him his inner being and its nature.

Finally, the existence of the *kundalini sense* may be revealed to people through an experience of *re-cognition* which is called up by some often trivial incident in the person's physical life that coincides with the memory of a former etheric experience or relationship. It sometimes manifests as a feeling of *déjà vu*. Nearly everyone has experienced, with varying degrees of sensitivity and awareness, a familiarity with people, places, or situations for which the known life cannot account. Many people experience strong affinities with a particular culture or language or music and art form which cannot be explained by the circumstances of their physical lives. A marked feeling of poignancy often accompanies these experiences, as if a former intimacy, once known and lost, were briefly touched again. Through his *kundalini sense* a person can receive many different indications of experiences and knowledge which *belong* to him through previous existence on etheric planes, and which are part of his etheric being. Through recognising their nature, the person builds new links between his present physical life and his real inner being.

III

After a person has taken the first steps in becoming aware of the *kundalini sense* in himself and its individual modes of expression, the next step lies in the Yoga practices of *savasana*. *Savasana* is concerned with the complete relaxation of body and mind and leads, ultimately, to states of mind called *meditation*, which is the attitude of listening or awareness that grows out of inner stillness. Relaxation of body and mind is a necessary preparation for growth in self-awareness; self-awareness is the first stage in meditation and precedes all other forms of awareness that extend gradually to include more and more of the etheric sphere in which the person has his being.

The first practice of *savasana* concerns relaxation of the body. A simple method is used, but for it to be effective it must be practised regularly, at least once a day for ten minutes, over a considerable period of time. The person proceeds in the following way: he lies on a mat on the floor, in a warm yet not airless place, and places his hands on his solar plexus. He gives attention first of all to his hands, then to his solar plexus and all the sensations connected with it. He seeks to be aware of it as the centre of his physical being, of its warmth, of the way in which it sends this sensation of warmth radiating out in all directions, to all parts of his body. As the person directs his attention to the solar plexus, he tries to relax all the muscles connected with it. When he has achieved what is possible for him at *that particular time*, he begins the relaxation of his whole body. In this, he commences with the feet and proceeds upwards, throughout the length of his body, tensing and relaxing each group of muscles in turn, as far as he can, and ending with the small muscles in his throat, tongue, face, and scalp. When he has achieved the degree of relaxation possible for him at that moment, he should continue to lie in this position for approximately three minutes.

When a person first commences this exercise of *savasana* he will find it difficult to apply his mind to giving attention in this way. He will also discover a low level of awareness in himself and tend to generalise and skip over whole groups or areas of muscle. In time, however, as he perseveres, he will become aware of greater detail and of the state of different sets of muscles. He will develop an awareness of the degrees of habitual tension existing in certain parts of his body. As he continues so lines of connection between these different physical tensions and certain habits of thought or thought-patterns will reveal themselves to him. When this begins to happen, he has reached the second stage in the practice of *savasana*.

With this new stage comes the need for an increased degree of mental relaxation and, with it, another level of awareness through which the person learns in greater detail about the inter-locking of his thought-patterns or attitudes of mind with muscle and body tension. At this stage the practice of *savasana* is extended into the person's daily life, and it is here that the inter-connections between mind and body are revealed to him most clearly – often as fleeting revelations in the middle of an experience or of instant 'photographs' impressed upon his mind. Awareness of a mental habit can recall a series of bodily tensions, or the experience of muscular contractions can call up a related thought-pattern. At this stage the person discovers that in order to relax the physical muscle he has to make a more conscious effort to release the related thought habit as well. This requires great patience and the will to persevere over a considerable period of time, for the inter-locking of thought-patterns and body tension has built-up through long association. These casual inter-relationships between mind and body have also created a structure of tensions in the person which is self-perpetuating. The activation, for example, of a particular muscular tension may evoke an anxiety-thought for no reason other than the fact of long association.

This second stage in the practice of *savasana* has to do with *loosening* the structure of inter-connected tensions and mental habits through relaxation, not of eradicating them. Any attempt at this point to eliminate tensions or their causes would either beget new ones or alter the form in which the old ones manifested. So the aim should not be directed to getting rid of tension – which would be another cause of tension – but rather to the relaxation of body and awareness of mind. But for relaxation and awareness to develop beyond their starting points, there must awaken in the person a willingness to proceed which is based on *acceptance*: an acceptance of what he observes to be his own mental and physical state at the time. The degree to which he accepts his state, or states, is a reflection of his own integrity, and upon this depend both his desire and ability to proceed with the practices of *savasana*.

Even in the beginning the practice of *savasana* can give a person temporary experiences of total relaxation; but the habitual patterns of mind will again be entered into and the old situations will call forth old tensions. However, they will not be quite the same, for something has happened as a result of *savasana*. The former state does not always return in the same form, nor with the same rigidity; old attitudes, and therefore former tensions, do not have the same hold on the person's mind. A new state of being is slowly developing through the practice of *savasana* which becomes in time like another room in the person's house of himself, into which he can learn to move at will and which he can eventually inhabit. But this is a further stage to which the person comes in time, as he proceeds with other forms of *savasana* which may loosely be called practices of *meditation*.

The experience of total relaxation, which has been described as 'another room' in the house of the person's being, is not an experience of emptiness but of completeness. His body is suffused with warmth and his mind is without tensions: he may seem to be 'floating';[23] and yet it is not the absence of tension which is most noticeable but the presence of something else. It is a state of harmony which reveals the presence of his own etheric being, his inner self.

The most 'active' factor in the etheric nature of a person[24] is called the Creative Imagination and is another name for the creative force within man's etheric being. It is not the same creative force[25] which created and maintains his physical body but rather his own unique ability to create, which is latent in every human being. Its direction and form are determined by each person's own will; its capacity for expression develops through usage and depends upon how and for what it is used. The Creative Imagination is the Divine creative faculty put into the being of everyone at the time of his spiritual creation. It has always been used by evolving beings to create the higher worlds of Light – and by distorted beings to create worlds where darkness and demons exist.

The Creative Imagination is expressed through man's physical being during his life in a physical body, its place of functioning being the central frontal part of the brain. It comes partly into the orbit of the physical mind and can be used by it, for the frontal part of man's brain is also the venue of his physical mind. This mind, as it develops, becomes connected with either the left or right frontal part of the brain – only one side of which is developed in any one person. (The whole of the frontal part of the brain is used by the self will.) All that a man creates, mentally and physically, during his physical lifetime is a result of the use his will makes of his Creative Imagination, which expresses through the agency of the physical mind. All spiritual growth in a man, at whatever stage, is first of all projected by his Creative Imagination as *potential* or as an outline of what is possible, *after which* it is 'entered into' and expressed by the man himself. The Creative Imagination makes the 'plan', as it were, which the man builds up through a continuing process of expression. But even the Creative Imagination does not *originate* anything new; all *new* creation, whether in the sense of a person's spiritual growth or his artistic expression, derives in seed form from a higher level of being outside the person himself. The Creative Imagination takes the 'seed' and works upon it. This is the principle on which each man's creation of himself is based; it describes the process by which he evolves slowly, over vast periods of time, and also the process of creation in that portion of the universe on which his life directly impinges and for which he is uniquely responsible.

All creation – apart from man – was created by the Creative Imagination of individual beings at various stages of evolution. Nothing exists which was not created in this way. The same Creative Imagination exists today in all men and, with it, infinite possibilities for further creation. But new creation is not, in fact, expressed only in the form of new stages in man's spiritual growth, but at every level and in ordinary daily existence in the personal world in which each individual lives and has his being. Every person uses his Creative Imagination from moment to moment to create the world in which he *really* lives, that is, the world through which he relates to everything in his life.[26]

Creation takes place, firstly, through the act of visualisation. In most people, visualisation is an activity that takes place in the head, through the Formatory or Physical Mind, the results of which are not complete 'creations' but *outlines of form* that become real to the person only through a process which requires a period of time. The process of making real what is initially an outline of form – that is, making subjectively real for the person himself – depends on the person's will and the degree of his willing. Thus, two activities are involved in most forms of creation, the act of visualisation and a process which commences with the act of willing. These two factors make up every human experience, for experience is creation.

This is the pattern of creation on the etheric plane, and every form which has – or is to have – physical shape is first of all an etheric manifestation. A building, a piece of sculpture, a painting, must be created etherically in every detail before it can be translated into stone and mortar, clay, or paint. This is the principle from which deviation is not possible.[27] A piece of music may even be heard *as a whole* by the inner ear of the composer before he comes to the stage of setting down the notation in time-sequence,[28] that is, creating its physical form.

All creation must take place first of all on the etheric plane; its translation into physical form – if it takes place at all – is the result of another process which is based on laws that govern all forms of expression on the physical earth. Most of creation exists only in etheric form, as etheric or spiritual reality for the person or persons concerned; it is not translated into physical form at all. All that men create through their physical minds constitutes etheric reality *for them*; this etheric world may not be expressed in physical form, and yet it affects and interpenetrates every aspect of a man's physical environment.

All creations that proceed from the Creative Imagination in a man are *real* and not abstract. Whatever the forms in which these creations are expressed, they have real existence for that person because they are composed of real etheric substance.

A man uses his Creative Imagination, consciously or unconsciously, according to the nature of his own being; he cannot do otherwise. It may manifest in hundreds of different ways in the everyday lives of people, for the Creative Imagination is the means by which the invisible or mental world is created within which most people on earth live most of their lives. It is only when someone has exhausted its possibilities in one direction or another, or tired of this 'world' within which he passes his life, that new possibilities of creation become open to him. When he comes to see the old forms of his creation as trivial or irrelevant or unreal, so his own Creative Imagination can offer an infinite response of new forms, according to the direction in which his will wishes to go and the Inspiration which he attracts. This Creative Imagination – the etheric Creative Force within all human beings – is always available when a man needs it, to create new forms of expression for the self and new worlds for him to inhabit.

But at certain stages, or when people are in a particular state, this Creative Imagination is often used to excite or overstimulate or titillate the senses, creating an exaggerated and highly-coloured world which can seriously distort the person's life. He may even come to depend upon this exaggerated world of fantasy and derive his meaning from it until it enters into all his relationships to others as well as to himself. This is the state of mind within which all forms of magic thrive and in which people are vulnerable to the apprehension of demons or to mental derangement. The private world of fantasy can lead a person into manifestation of mass hysteria at political rallies or football matches and religious forms of emotionalism, such as speaking in tongues. It is the power of the Creative Imagination in people to which demagogues or wartime leaders appeal and which they draw on to create mass states of mind. To this faculty in man, and under certain conditions or in certain states, is due the appeal of such varied public displays as Roman Circuses, public executions, Royal Weddings, and Disneylands. It can be used as a source of exaggeration and unreason on mass scale to give people a sense of importance through participating in events or crises or fantasy worlds.

This highly-coloured world which people can create for themselves at certain stages, and in which they are to themselves the centre, is *real* for them and they usually attract other people into their lives who share in the same kind of 'reality'. But it has only subjective validity and is not real in itself; it has no objective reality.

In time, this 'world' within which a person lives his life – whatever its meanings, fantasies, or distractions – is revealed to him for what it is. Understanding comes gradually and new truths are disclosed again and again as the person is slowly loosened from the 'pictures' of himself and his life which his mind had created. But at each stage a man loses only what has already, in a sense, ceased to exist for him. It may be replaced immediately by another picture of his life, with only slight alterations in the former structure of his mind. In this case, no space intervenes between the two states, but one interior world slowly merges into the other. In some cases, where the person is making real spiritual growth, the world he created, and in which he lived, is replaced temporarily with a desert-like world where he experiences greater clarity of vision and understanding about the nature of these pictures and the structure of what he had previously taken as reality. However brief such an experience may be, the *quality* of 'truth' changes for him and never returns to its previous state. For an individual's 'truth' derives from his experience and the state of his being; it is the essence of *what he takes as real.* Occasionally he may have an insight into that other Truth which is more complex and many-facetted than anything of which he could have conceived previously. For Truth – all-embracing, Objective Truth – is *an experience* of the total and evolving world, with all its levels of being, at any single moment of existence.

One task of the person who has entered upon an experience of 'desert' or 'wilderness' is to identify the elements of fantasy or unreality in his life, which had placed limitations upon his own spiritual growth; the second task is to experience what is *now*. Fantasy of one kind or another has prevented the person living in *now*. He has lived to a certain extent in what was going to happen next or, retrospectively, in past experiences. This is imaginary as far as the *now-ness* of things is concerned.

It is very difficult to experience *now*. The experience of *now* may seem empty and even dull to someone whose mind has seldom been still or who has rarely taken in 'what is' because the mind he had created was always there to colour or re-structure it – to distract him from it or in some way to impose its own pattern upon it. *Now* seems colourless and insipid because the person is more used to artificial colour or artificial stimulants.

To live in the present – the *now* – requires a conscious effort. And it is largely through various practices of meditation[29] that the person develops states of awareness which make this possible. These practices are discussed in detail in a later section, and belong in theory to the stage of *pratyahara*; but in fact the practice of meditation begins much earlier for the student of Yoga, whenever the need arises in him, and develops in different forms throughout every stage of his evolution.

Dreamlike states and fantasy-dominated worlds exist on subconscious levels where little or no effort is required and a person may, in a certain sense, drift through his life.[30] Such states can slowly fade as the person's awareness grows, for they are semi-automatic. The purpose inherent in the effort required to recognise the different elements of fantasy which structure the life of a person is to bring him to a higher state of consciousness in which he has a more continuous awareness of himself and his life. All states of awareness make possible at least some distinction between subjective and objective reality and permit new forms of experience. From being the victim of a subconscious dreamlike existence, the person can progress through stages of seeing and experiencing things more nearly *as they are* and come to the stage in his evolution where he is master in his own house, to a certain extent, and able to control the mind which would distort and weave its web of fantasy around his life.

But to begin with he has to see and accept the reality of his own self will, as it is, and the subjective fantasy world which this will has created and out of which it seeks to act upon every situation around him. He has to accept the inability of his own will to act in relation to situations *without* fantasy or without the desire to alter them.[31] When the person can accept his own limitations and the inability of his will to act *non*-subjectively, he begins to make contact with part of his own etheric being which can inspire him with the knowledge that eventually makes a different kind of action possible.

If a person is to accept his daily life he has to accept the realities in his life as they are: the people, the conditions, and the events as they occur. This involves, in part, acknowledging his inability to alter factors which are unalterable. A decrease in the need to alter the conditions of his life gives rise to less dissatisfaction. When the man is more contented and less agitated and excitable, through desire for superficial change, so the real possibility of altering *some* things begins to arise. The possibility of real change derives from the man's etheric being and not from his self will. With growth in awareness, there develops in the person an increasing desire to take responsibility for his own life and to have more control over his own body and mind. In this way opportunities occur for the kind of change consonant with spiritual reality.

If a person can accept all that occurs in his everyday life, the power of the self will is lessened and he becomes more open to the *kundalini sense* and the possibility of re-establishing contact with his own etheric being.

Acceptance is a conscious act. It requires a considerable degree of awareness, for example, to accept interruptions as events that belong to a particular day; to curb an habitual impatience with someone through accepting the reality of that person's nature, which only he can alter; to say 'yes' to an activity which is usually performed with reluctance and recognise its place in the structure of the daily life.

Acceptance also means a conscious saying of 'yes' to the unalterable circumstances and conditions within which the person's own life is set, which have outwardly structured his life, or which form the social-cultural web within which his life is expressed.

Wasteful in energy and damaging to the person's relationship to *himself* is his failure to accept the structure of conditions or circumstances into which he was personally born. Parents, education, and social status can be used by anyone to justify his failure to make spiritual effort – to justify his own laziness – and enable him to postpone the commencement of the kind and degree of spiritual growth which would be right for him at a particular stage. So long as a person in any way rejects the personal circumstances which form – or formed – the external structure of his life, so long will his attention be directed away from the purpose for which he came into this life, and so long will he be looking to *external* conditions to provide solutions and securities.

Each person attracts his own set of circumstances according to his own etheric being, its nature, and the stage of its evolution. It is only from *where he is* that a person can begin to grow spiritually, and 'where he is' means the kind of being he has developed, with all its strengths and weaknesses, up to the time of his entrance into physical life. It is both logical and essential that the *external* circumstances of his physical life should reflect in some degree the vibrations of his own real etheric nature.[32] Therefore, growth in a person's being can only commence when he has turned around from the attitude that sees *causes* in external circumstances and has begun to use them instead to show him something of the nature of his own being; for these circumstances suggest – at least in part – the purpose for which he came into a physical life.

This is particularly important with regard to a person's parents.

Whoever they are, or whatever their relationship to him at any particular stage, his own growth of being depends upon an acceptance of them *as they are* and the fact of his relationship to them. 'Blame of parents' is an effective obstacle to any kind of growth in a person.

The present physical life of every person is the only possible starting point for his spiritual growth. All that belongs to the person's mental or manual equipment is *his own* and belongs to no one else in exactly the same form, for it has been earned previously by his own efforts. As no two people make identical effort in their etheric lives, so no two people will have identical equipment to use in their physical lives[33] – or identical weaknesses. Each person's physical life – its circumstances, conditions, and relationships – is his own particular field of work in relation to which his etheric nature and character can develop and grow. He alone has the task and the ability to work his own 'field', which is the segment of Life that belongs to him alone.

IV

Since before the time of Patanjali, at least two thousand years ago, the section or step in yoga called *pranayama* has meant solely 'control of the breath' or exercises by which a man stopped, held, or punctuated his breathing for purposes which were only in part physiological. The ultimate aim of all breath control, as taught by traditional yoga schools, is mind control and the creation of certain states of being. In the original oral teaching of Yoga, however, breathing exercises as such occupied only a small part of the subject of *pranayama* and were taught solely for physiological reasons. No controls were ever placed on the inhalation or exhalation of the breath itself nor were any artificial rhythms imposed on the motion of the lungs. The later practice of breath-stoppages was never taught in this earliest form of Yoga because it had no connection with the purpose implicit in the breathing exercises which was the development of health and balance in the natural physical man. Breath-control would have been considered dangerous as an interference with natural physiological processes; for only slight physical benefit would result from such exercises, and they could damage the ability of the lungs to perform their natural function.

Detailed breathing exercises, involving both control and stoppage of the breath, were invented by priests and formed part of temple or religious practices at a later time – beginning about a thousand years after the oral teaching of Yoga commenced. They are recorded briefly in the *Yoga Aphorisms of Patanjali*; in a simple, more innocuous form, they constitute part of the Yoga-for-Health teaching of the West. They were developed originally for the purpose of attaining to abnormal (or supra-normal) states of consciousness and acquiring certain psychic powers. As such, these breathing techniques became part of a vast body of diverse religious and philosophical teachings whose narrow and distorted practices may be found in some measure in every religious or quasi-religious group all over the world. All such practices become in the end an obstacle to man's real spiritual development because they interfere with the *normal* functioning of his physical and mental being upon which his spiritual development depends. Spiritual growth can only be gradual. To attempt short-cuts, of whatever nature, sets up inner blockages and distortions which may take a long time to remove or remedy before the person can enter again upon his true spiritual journey.

In the original oral teaching of Yoga two different kinds of exercise were taught – and are still being taught – in connection with *pranayama*. For physiological purposes, the *Full Yoga Breath* was taught as the principal breathing technique to expand the lungs to their full capacity; in this connection pupils learned about the importance of fully oxygenating the blood-stream to keep the body's cells and tissue in good repair and to release toxic matter. They were given enough knowledge about the nature and functioning of their own bodies for them to be able to understand the importance of having a regular and sufficient supply of oxygen to maintain the body in a state of health. In the twentieth century, this Full Yoga Breath is of even greater relevance than it was five or six thousand years ago – in fact, its importance can scarcely be exaggerated if a man's body is to remain (or even become) healthy; for the habits of shallow breathing and hollow chests, impure air, and the greatly increased incidence of toxic matter (particularly in the form of chemicals) in man's body have been in large part responsible for his present state of physical disharmony. This state did not exist, or only rarely, in earlier times. Hence, the increased importance of teaching the Full Yoga Breath to twentieth century man before going on to the series of *pranayama* exercises.

The Full Yoga Breath commences with the student standing or lying – *never* sitting – in a relaxed position. He first of all becomes aware of his Solar Plexus and begins a slow in-take of breath as if it were being drawn into the Solar Plexus. He allows the breath to rise, on a slow rhythmical count, through the lower, middle, and upper lungs. As breath fills his lungs so he extends his arms up and out to increase their capacity. When the lungs are full, there is no pause and the breath is slowly released, on the same slow rhythmical count, and leaves the upper, middle, and lower lungs in that order, the arms being lowered simultaneously. The student practises this two or three times a day, taking a minimum of four Full Yoga Breaths on each occasion.

The second kind of exercise connected with *pranayama* is not a breathing exercise in the strictest sense, because the student is not in fact directing the *breath* at all. In every form of this exercise it is the *rhythm* of inhaling and exhaling air which is used as a focus for drawing in Creative Force. These exercises are an essential part of the teaching about *pranayama* because they have to do with the individual's *practice* in learning to have control over the Creative Force. The essence of each exercise lies not in the act of breathing but in the absorption of 'free' *prana* and the directing of this and the internal Creative Force (that is, the Creative Force inherent in the person himself) to various parts of the body to cleanse or clear away toxins and other waste matter, or to heal.[34]

In performing this exercise of *pranayama* the person visualises drawing the Creative Force into the centre of Elimination on an inhaled breath and directing it to the part or parts of his body in need of cleansing or re-vitalising. In order to be effective, this must be repeated continuously for a period of five minutes. This is the pattern for all the exercises of *pranayama*.

Every exercise of *pranayama* is based on a relaxed, easy rhythm of breathing which is neither shallow nor deep but performed slowly and without strain. Once established, the rhythm of breathing must be natural and require no conscious effort, for the person should be able to give his whole attention to the directing of *prana*.

There are eight specific exercises of *pranayama* apart from the general cleansing exercise given above. Seven of these exercises follow the same basic pattern, commencing with the person placing his consciousness in each of the seven centres in turn. 'Placing his consciousness' means visualising the particular centre in terms of its position on the spine, its meaning, and its function, and then *entering into it*, as it were, so that the person feels he is inhabiting it. From his consciousness in that centre, however limited it may be, he visualises drawing in *prana* or the Creative Force (while he simultaneously and slowly draws in his breath). Visualising means not so much 'seeing' as the use of all his senses in an *interior* way to 'feel' or 'experience' the drawing in of *prana* into a particular centre. This involves considerable use of his Creative Imagination. Thoughts will possibly occur to the man as to the nature of *prana*; in fact, a person may be sensitive to many aspects of the *prana* nature while performing this exercise. He may also experience a sense of wonder or mystery. As the person draws *prana* into a particular centre, he should have in mind that the reason for doing so is to cleanse, heal, and strengthen that centre. Finally, on the exhaled breath – and there should be no pause or holding of the breath – the person visualises the dispersal of anything which might impede the perfect functioning of the particular centre. The exercise is repeated five times for each centre, that is, with five complete breaths.

This exercise may be performed for one centre only or it may be taken as a seven-fold exercise in which each centre is focussed on in turn. In the seven-fold exercise, the person commences with the three lower centres – the order is not important, but he should take time and care to become conscious in each one before performing *pranayama*. This means that the person should truly 'centre himself' in each *chakra* and experience its nature before beginning the exercise connected with that centre. After performing the exercise of *pranayama* in the lower three centres, he proceeds to the Solar Plexus, then to the Heart, Throat, and Head Centres, following the same procedure with each one.

These seven exercises – or the seven-fold exercise – must always precede the eighth exercise which has to do with drawing *prana* up and down the spine, from the Sex Centre to the Head Centre. This final exercise of *pranayama* is an important exercise, for it joins the whole being of a man together by connecting the seven centres with one another. Six of these centres are situated on the spinal column of the invisible physical body of man and reflected onto his physical spinal column; the seventh, or Head Centre, is sited above the spinal column, so there is a gap between it and the spinal column which contains the other six centres. There is a definite purpose in this gap. The Head Centre is separated from all the other centres so that it can have the innate capacity for functioning independently and be able to inspire or direct a man, whatever his stage of evolution, from outside the limits of his physical life and experience. Separated from the other centres in this way, the Head Centre is free to receive and channel knowledge which belongs to the person from previous experiences of an etheric nature and which is contained within his etheric being.

The main purpose of the eighth exercise of *pranayama* is to relate all seven centres in a man to one another and to create a functioning *whole*. An important aspect of this lies in bridging the gap between the spinal column and the Head Centre and thus bring the inspirations coming from that centre into relationship with the other six centres.

The exercise is performed in this way. On an intake of breath the person visualises *prana* entering his spine at the Sex Centre and travelling up one side of it, through each of the other centres: Elimination and Digestion Centres, Solar Plexus, Heart, Throat, and Head Centres. As *prana* travels up the spine, he should make the effort to *feel himself* briefly into each centre in turn, visualising its nature and purpose. At the Head Centre he 'turns around', as it were, and brings *prana* down the other side of the spine, through the centres in reverse order, as he exhales his breath. On the succeeding complete breath he brings *prana* up the other side of the spine and down the first side, thus alternating sides in the up-and-down movement of *prana* for five complete breaths.

All eight exercises have the purpose of cleansing, healing, and strengthening the centres and the channels in the spine[35] through which the centres are connected with one another in the invisible physical body. The cleansing is necessary because of abnormal ways in which man lives his life on earth, feeding his mind and body on what can cause distortion or malfunctioning. Only when the centres are functioning correctly in themselves is the harmonious working together of them possible which was intended for man's physical life on earth.

These exercises also help to develop those centres which have remained under-developed through the way in which a man has lived in his physical body[36] and to so adjust their working that each centre is able to perform its true function[37] and not usurp that of another centre. The exercises also serve the very important purpose of making the person more aware of the centres in himself and of the underlying unity of being which their functioning should reflect. As his consciousness increases of both the existence and the harmonious working of all his centres, so they *in fact* begin to work in approximation to the true potential which they had when he was first born into a physical body.[38]

All people come into a physical life with etheric beings which are in some state of imbalance in one direction or another, because all development is one-sided and has to do with first one aspect of a man's being and then another. A man's centres are, however, not only unequal in relation to their inherent potentialities, but their ability to function normally is distorted by the way in which man lives his life on the physical earth. This kind of distortion is very different from the basic etheric imbalance which exists in everyone in some degree – and is very exaggerated in some people. In part, the distortion caused by man's life on the physical earth is due to his self will which identifies more with one function than another and may create a structure of fantasy around its activities. These fantasies have been rationalised by theorists in all ages but in particular by twentieth century psychologists who develop theories about the personality or psychological 'types of man' – categories into which all people are supposed to fall because of innate differences.[39] These may, in fact, be kinds of imbalance which belong to a certain stage in the person's evolution or they may represent kinds of distortion characteristic of a particular society or culture at any one time. These limited and often irrelevant explanations of human psychology tend to encourage people to continue with their self fantasies, giving them theories to justify the labels they pin on themselves. The initial imbalance in a person can be strengthened in this way; his centres may remain under-developed or their functioning may even atrophy or become distorted in the direction emphasized by the particular theory.

The eight exercises of *pranayama* can begin to rectify this situation more effectively than could be done by any other means, because they unite the efforts of a man's consciousness, will, Creative Imagination, and physical being. They give him actual *experience* of the different centres, their functioning and relationships to one another, and of that unity in which all the functions form a whole within his own personal being.

All the centres in individual men and women have certain potentials for working which differ from person to person, the potential in any one man being the result of his previous spiritual efforts before entering physical life. These potentials vary in accordance with the stages people have reached in their spiritual development; but however undeveloped spiritually the being of a person may be, it nonetheless contains all seven centres. No one on earth is entirely without the intuitive faculty of the Head Centre or the ability to communicate in some form or other through the Throat Centre. It is a dangerous abstraction which suggests that one person or another is not an intuitive type. He doesn't know about his intuitions, he doesn't hear them, perhaps; but this doesn't mean that they are not functioning to some extent in every person on earth.

A man does not need to make effort in order to develop those functions in himself which are under-developed. In fact, the actual making of effort and the person's *motive* in doing so may create a further imbalance and divert him from a growth pattern which would manifest and evolve naturally in relation to his own growth in awareness. For his first task is to extend his awareness of himself gradually beyond the artificial pictures he has of himself. He has to become aware of and observe his centres through the practices of *pranayama* without criticism. As he focusses his attention on each one of the centres in turn, he holds in his mind a conception of the true nature and function of the centre and of any malfunctioning or weakness of which he is aware. As he does this, and as he performs the exercises, he will become aware of a change gradually taking place. He will be aware of a stronger, more assured and responsive working of the centre and of distortions slowly diminishing. These real – physical and conscious – experiences of his own centres and their working will give the person greater confidence in his own being; they will also act on his acquired or artificial attitudes and ideas about himself and bring about gradually a loosening of their influence over his mind.

The experience of these *pranayama* exercises will also allow the natural unity of a person's being,[40] as it should have existed at birth,[41] gradually to become part of his own consciousness. He will have an increasing *experience* of wholeness,[42] not merely an *idea about* the unity of his being. He will experience the various functions that belong to both the physical and etheric parts of his being as they are at his own stage of evolution, and his understanding of their natures in relation to one another will deepen through inspiration. It is only this *experience* of the nature and wholeness of his own being, the growing sense of confidence which it can generate, and the consequent ability to assume responsibility for his own life that form the basis for any real change in a person and are the foundation for all spiritual growth.

True teaching relates only to what men are able at each stage to *experience* for themselves; it never has to do with abstract knowledge or theories which are not relevant or in some way related to a man's own understanding, at different stages. All true teaching must also be based upon the experience of the *whole* man and include every aspect of his etheric *and* physical being. Any teaching which is partial and creates dualisms or attempts to exclude one part of man's being or experience, with the intention of improving or strengthening another part, is a false teaching because it seeks to create an artificial man; it does not start from the natural man or from the man's true nature or reality. These two criteria are useful measures against which to examine the validity of teachers and teachings.

V

When the *kundalini sense* begins to function in a person, at whatever stage in his life, and he is re-connected in some degree with his previous etheric experiences – although he may be wholly unaware of what is happening,[43] a certain amount of energy is released in him. This new source of energy finds expression in whatever direction the will is facing at the moment of its release. If the person is still dominated by self fantasies of which he is unconscious, this new energy will go to increase their power over him. Often the accession of new energy makes a person feel more powerful and it goes into those forms through which his desire to experience power have been expressed.

The desire for the experience of power exists in men from the beginning, for it belongs to the nature of man's will, and is expressed on all the lower stages in etheric life as well as through the physical lives of men on earth. It is centred in his Sex Centre, which is the focal point for his feeling of 'I'; but it does not belong exclusively to man's physical nature or to his physical life. In fact, it is part of his etheric being and expresses in various forms throughout the first four levels of his evolution until, after very long periods of time, a man has evolved beyond the fourth level and no longer seeks his own identity through an experience of power. But until a person has evolved to this point, the desire for power exists in one form or another in him and he is vulnerable to the dangers or distractions which it opens him up to, whether he lives in a physical or etheric body.

The desire for the experience of power has many different forms of expression, depending upon the person's previous experiences, the particular direction his life has taken, and the historical epoch and cultural milieu to which he has been attracted and in which his physical life is expressed.

Power-seeking manifests most obviously in the practice of magic. Various forms of the practice of magic have existed in all ages and cultures (and continue to exist in etheric spheres, for they do not belong exclusively to the physical earth). Some of these forms are simple and uncomplicated, being expressions of the day-to-day existence of less sophisticated people in their relationships to the material, visible, and invisible world around them. These forms are generally innocuous and have little damaging or lasting effect on their minds. More sophisticated forms, developed by people with either complex or distorted beings, can do more damage; and intellectualised expressions of the desire for power, which are reinforced by complicated structures of rationalisation, can damage or distort the whole etheric being of a person. Such damage may extend far beyond his earth experience and can take centuries of earth-time to eradicate.

The desire for the experience of power can also take the form of the desire *to be possessed by power*. In modern times this often finds expression in the seeking for individual identity through group or mass power – although the desire to participate in expressions of group power has always existed, in one form or another. At all times in human history a person's desire to participate in a power experience[44] (as distinct from his desire to possess power or instruments of power for himself) has meant in fact a relinquishment of his own will and an opening up of his being to allow the will of another to enter in to use or possess him.[45] Not that the true nature and structure of this experience is recognised or understood by the person or persons concerned. Different interpretations are given and various theories advanced on the subject of power possession and the desire to be possessed by power, but the fact is that the desire in a person for this *kind* of experience sends out a vibration which is a form of invitation to those in the spirit world who await such opportunities for expression. The concept that such power is impersonal or resides solely in the person himself only increases the potential danger; against such possession he can see no need for protection.

The idea of the existence of a kundalini *force* derived originally from the experience of being possessed by power. This theory was constructed by a small cult within the Hindu religions, several hundred years before the time of Buddha, by men who desired above all else the experience of power-possession and who, through experimentation on themselves, had worked out techniques for opening their beings to what was, in fact, *spirit*-possession. These people had no understanding of what they were doing. They imagined that the kundalini force was a power to be awakened in themselves, which could be increased from impersonal power sources in the universe, and that this could be achieved through the techniques they had devised. Furthermore, they were not aware of the nature of their motives, which were both personal and 'group' in origin; for along with their obsession with personal power-possession was the desire to increase and spread the power of their own sect. Through the elaboration of such a theory, devised and taught by their own sect, they alone would act as its interpreters, they alone would instruct people and lead them to an awakening of the same kundalini force in themselves. They alone would be the arbiters of who should be allowed to awaken this force in himself and under what conditions, and who should not. But of these underlying motives they were, at that time, unaware. The theory of the kundalini force evolved through the years, taking on more refinements, increasing sophistication, various interpretations.

All theories regarding a kundalini force are based on certain facts about the nature of man.[46] The principal set of facts used in these theories relates to the structure of the spine in man's invisible physical body and the three channels it contains, which are a central channel and two connected channels that form a continuous oval around it. The two channels are in fact used by the Creative Force in each person for the purpose of maintaining or healing the person's invisible physical body and, through it, his physical body. These channels are essential for the maintenance of a man's health during his life in a physical body. The central channel is used solely to transmit the basic energy-substance, that derives from each person's individual will, to the separate *chakras*, or centres, where it is transformed into the different types of energy required by these centres for their functioning. All energy-substance in a man derives originally from his will but is developed for use by the different centres into separate forms of energy. Energies are developed in a man's *invisible* physical body but are drawn on for the functioning of his physical body and for every activity in which it is engaged during his physical life on earth.

The basic energy-substance in one man differs from that in every other person; no two energy-substances are ever the same, any more than two individual wills are ever identical. The nature of this energy-substance, and the various forms in which it is developed by the centres in a man, remains consistent and in accordance with the nature of his will regardless of changes in his health, mood, desires, life-pattern, etc. Only one factor can alter the nature of a man's basic energy-substance and that is a change in the level of his being or in the degree of his consciousness. A man's consciousness becomes transformed with the evolution of his will; as the nature of his will evolves in direction and structure so his energy-substance becomes finer and more adaptable. These finer vibrations affect the working of his seven centres. This is the *true* change which can be effected by the only force that vibrates through the central channel in man's spine, and such change is *only* possible with the growth in his awareness, consciousness, and being.

The theories that relate to a kundalini force are also based on the actual existence of a certain substance of which the people who propound these theories are completely unaware. This is an etheric substance which was constructed by certain individuals in spirit form for the *destruction* of mankind and all his creative achievements. This destructive substance was 'created' around the beginning of the third millenium B.C. by persons who had acquired certain powers during their lifetimes in the so-called Old Kingdom of Egypt and who extended and made use of these powers for evil purposes after their physical death. One result was the creation of this destructive substance, which has been used ever since that time by certain individuals in spirit form whose purpose was to break up or destroy every kind of living or non-living form on both the etheric and physical planes. This was to be achieved by using the destructive substance to over-excite or increase the rate of vibration of people's nervous systems, or the structures of any animal or plant, or the composition of an inanimate, material form.

All living or inanimate forms can be affected by this destructive substance on the physical plane; but on the etheric plane only human beings can be affected by it. This substance is never *impersonal* and can never affect any form of life or any object except when it is deliberately used by a person or persons.[47] Knowledge about its existence belongs primarily to people on etheric planes, and its systematic use to destroy all that men create and to distract them from their spiritual journeys originates in the lowest and darkest spheres of the etheric world.

All theories that postulate a kundalini force encourage the opening up of individuals to an excitement of their beings or an over-stimulation of their nervous systems through what they imagine to be the entrance of this desirable kundalini force. In fact, it is an invitation to those in spirit form who seek to destroy, and what is naively imagined to be the kundalini force is actually the destructive substance.

At its commencement, over-excitement always appears to be a kind of energy – and, in a certain sense it is, for the feeling of power coincides with a new thrust of energy that derives from the person or persons using this substance of destruction. Any increase in energy always comes from *outside* the man who is affected by this destructive substance and is the personal energy of the ones who seek to destroy. *Every* increase in the quantity of energy within a person always derives from outside his own being. Additional energy therefore makes the person increasingly dependent upon those from whom the energy derives so that even his own will is ultimately affected. The over-stimulation of the nervous system brings about its deterioration in time and a degeneration in the structure of that person's body, the rate of decline being related to the intrinsic nature of the person. The brain of a person is the first part affected by any increase in vibration, and it becomes increasingly difficult for the person to give attention, or concentrate, or even remain normally sensitive to the world around him. Eventually all the organs in his body can be affected by over-stimulation.

It is important to realise that this destructive substance cannot enter the being of a person or animal, or into any inanimate form, unless there is the will to destroy. Will is always personal, and the will to destroy life and form is always the will of an individual person. The word 'evil' describes this will to destroy or any person's act of willing destruction. The inherent meaning of *evil* is exactly this, namely, the will to destroy what is divine or what has been created for the purpose of man's spiritual growth; the word 'evil' does not refer to the substance itself, which was built up by those who willed evil but which has no active power in itself.

Everything within a person that leads him to desire or enjoy the experience of participation in power, or of power-possession, is directly opposed to man's spiritual and conscious growth, for it proceeds from his fantasies about self; it is also an invitation to control – or possession – from outside, with the result that his degree of awareness is lessened, his own will is over-shadowed by another will, and his sense of personal responsibility is diminished. Such a man becomes an open channel through which any discarnate spirit, or spirits, can express, either temporarily or over a longer period of time. In most cases the man will not be conscious of what is happening, but will experience merely a new rush of power or an increase of force behind some form of self expression or sometimes a wave of emotion violently expressing through him. All this he takes as 'I', usually enjoying the more extreme feeling of himself – even if its expression is occasionally violent, but never suspecting its origin. The dangers to his own being can scarcely be exaggerated.

So long as a man desires power, whether consciously or unconsciously, so long will he be open to possession by unseen spirits of a kind which is far more dangerous to himself and others than are those forms of discarnate spirit possession which occur temporarily in the lives of the majority of people on earth today.[48] For a large proportion of people are not only open to temporary forms of spirit possession, through moods reflective of inherent weaknesses, but they bring with them, through under-developed or distorted beings, some unresolved personal attachment from their previous existence on etheric planes. Such negative attachments often take on a form of spirit possession during the physical life which cannot be resolved until that life is ended. It is not these forms of possession which are of the greatest danger to the person and those about him, but the ones which occur in the course of the man's physical life as a direct result of his desire for power.

The first danger is to the man's own being and the influence his desire for the experience of power can gradually acquire over it, his mind becoming re-structured in relation to the forms his desire takes. Through these forms discarnate spirits establish a pattern of entrance and possession. So long as the person continues in this desire for the experience of power, so long will this pattern remain set. All spiritual growth ceases, and his being can begin to grow again only after the desire for power has worked itself out and the structure of mind been broken down which it had built up. This state can last throughout the whole of his physical life and for a period of time following his life on earth.

The second kind of danger exists for other people with whom this person is connected and through whom their minds may become damaged in certain respects. This damage is never lasting – although it can remain with a person for the whole of his physical life – and can easily be remedied at the conclusion of that life on earth. Nevertheless, the *natural* pattern of his earth-life is altered and may even become distorted.

A third form of danger exists for the discarnate spirits themselves who have become caught up with the person's desire for the experience of power. If they become involved in only a *temporary* expression of emotion through the physical being of someone, or if they merely continue to express their own forms of identification with former earth-experience *without* doing this through the physical beings of other people, their own period of bondage is not unnecessarily protracted. These spirits are open to various forms of help which the spirit world (as well as certain people on the physical earth) can offer, and learning and change of being proceed steadily and naturally for them. However, when discarnate spirits become involved in more permanent forms of possession, the task of freeing them is made much more difficult. For one thing, the desire of the spirits to possess is linked with that of the man who is possessed, and this bond grows in strength as all concerned – the one in a physical body and the ones who are discarnate – become increasingly interlocked in a complex structure from which it may take a long period of work to extricate them. All the people who form part of this structure of possession are affected and the *natural* expression of their minds and beings is suspended until such time as this structure is broken down.

Another aspect of the desire for power finds expression in and through religious institutions and their systems of mythology and rationalisation. As these institutions grow so they become vast systems in which all the people involved feel bound together or secured[49] through *belief* in their redemptive power or the meaning their lives derive through belonging and participation. This structure of formalised inter-relationship, in which peoples' lives interlock with one another, is secured by the articles of belief and the rituals upon which any particular religious institution is founded and which subconsciously threaten the person who deviates or seeks to think independently with 'hell-fire' as well as with social ostracism. The real danger for the etheric being of a person whose life is involved in a religious institution lies in the hold it exerts over his mind which projects far beyond the lifetime of the physical body.

The people for whom all religious institutions present the greatest danger are its own priests and acolytes whose lives are inextricably interwoven with them. Through the church or temple, moreover, the server experiences power over other people – and power on an even vaster scale through his role or position in it. This is the sense of power which the church or institution and its systems of belief lend him by way of being able to confer or withhold the blessings of forgiveness, healing, peace, absolution. Also, in all systems of belief (philosophical and political as well as religious) is incorporated a hierarchy of 'demons', power over which a priest has in varying degrees – in some instances through the ritual of exorcism.

The danger for the person involved in such a system exists in the extent to which it closes the door on any free expression of his own being, through which eventually he has to grow and learn, as well as on the direction of spiritual growth which his being would *naturally* follow. If the church or system rejects the forms of expression natural to his own spiritual growth, as it must do in time by its very nature as an institution or *system* of beliefs, the person will seldom be able even to recognise what is natural to his own being and its growth or, recognising it, break away from the all-embracing structure of belief in which he finds himself. The fact of belonging to a religion or system of beliefs makes such an act of independence almost impossible for a person, because his entire future life or salvation seems to him to depend upon his continuing adherence to it. Independence of thought is not only heretical but, in terms of every system, a rejection of both salvation and the spiritual goal towards which the person is striving.[50] Long periods of help from outside – from the spiritual realms and from those in physical bodies who are qualified to assist – are necessary before the person can truly be freed from the hold which a church or system of belief exercises over his being.

The story of the man who sells his soul to the Devil exists in all ancient legends and tales. The Devil represents what the man desires most to possess – but which ends up by possessing him. In each person this comes back to the desire for power in some form: the power of magic, mystical power, sexual power, or the more sophisticated forms of power by which a man can rationalise his own being to himself and know he is 'right'. Ultimately, each man's Devil is created by his imagination about himself; whatever its form, it both serves and feeds this imagination, developing it, justifying it, and thereby increasing its power over the person. A state of fear also gives power to a man's Devil, and, conversely, the Devil increases a man's fear; for fear is the ultimate expression of his inability to accept reality and can only flourish where a mind is founded on fantasy.

The Devil may be defined as the power of imagination and self fantasies over a person. Anything which increases or feeds this power may be said to be 'in league with the Devil'. Even where the results may be of benefit to other people, as, for example, in the performance of spirit healing, if there is any sensation of power to feed the person's image of self or give him a sense of identity, the activity may be referred to as the 'work of the Devil'.[51] A few positive results can never justify causing distortion in the being of the person through whom these results come; and, in the end, the distorting influence of the imagination about the self, and the desire for power to feed it, will make itself felt even through healing vibrations, as they extend to other people. *Whatever* the nature of an activity,[52] if it encourages what is imaginary or distorted in the person, it can only in the end reflect distortion onto all the other people involved.

Magical practices constitute the most obvious expressions of power, magic being the naked use of any form of power by the self and the self absorbed will. The distinction between so-called white magicians and black magicians is not fundamental: *all* magicians desire and use power for themselves, whether the results for other people are good or bad. Their *motives* may be different – and this does distinguish magicians from one another. The black magician intends to do harm and wills it; the white magician intends to do good but is unconscious of what is involved and so does harm to himself and often to others as well. The results for all magicians have the effect of strengthening the hold of imagination upon the mind and increasing the taste for and enjoyment of power. Even the healer may be a magician, however good or true the results obtained. And in the long run a healer-magician can affect many lives adversely because of his often hidden motive of power-seeking which gives rise to jealousy, envy, and, often, bitter disappointment.

There are certain characteristic ways in which the power of imagination manifests in people who are dominated by it or which point unmistakably to this state of being. (a) The person whose life centres around the power of imagination is usually in a state of abundant or exaggerated good health through which he or she tends to dominate people who are physically weaker. This is always accompanied by insensitivity to the states of others. The person can eat what he likes and even do what he likes with impunity for a long time, careless of the energy supply which seems limitless and often deliberately insulting to the more careful husbanding of resources which other people need to employ. (b) There is often a noticeable neglect of personal and daily responsibilities, except where they form part of the structure of his fantasies about self. (c) The person's mind always contains a number of rigid attitudes which, when challenged, reveal their power over the person in the violence of his reaction. (d) There is also a strong flavour of sexuality in the person's obsession with some aspect of self which is particularly apparent in all forms of religiosity, mysticism, spiritualistic and occult expressions, healing and allied gifts, and in certain artistic expressions. This is often projected outwards onto an object – healer, teacher, god – as onto a lover. Much poetry of the Christian mystics bears witness to this, as do some parts of Church liturgy. This is not normal sexuality but the result of the power of imagination over a person. Behind it, driving that imagination, is a power which derives ultimately from some form of possession or inter-penetration by the spirit world.

The structure of all forms of fanaticism and obsession can be understood only in terms of this fact, that the excessive power behind these forms derives, without exception, from discarnate spirits. Discarnate spirits express through people's own weaknesses. These weaknesses are of different kinds and may be of inertia or despondency, anger or jealousy; they may derive from an imbalance in the person's being due to lack of development in certain directions or from attitudes originating in undigested pre-earth experiences. Discarnate spirits working through some weaknesses may lead the person to severe mental illness or even to acts of violence. Psychiatric hospitals and prisons in modern times are full of people whose personal weaknesses have been used and expressed through by large numbers of discarnate spirits who are themselves still trapped in their own weaknesses and in the desire to continue to express them.

People can become trapped in various forms of frustration, depression, bitterness, or fear. These states, like all strongly negative states, attract from the invisible etheric planes surrounding the person like-minded discarnate spirits who reinforce the person's state with their own. This kind of unfortunate relationship can imprison both persons more deeply in the negative states which brought about the initial connection. It can last far beyond the physical lifetime.

A similar negative link can be formed through an act of violence in which both assailant and victim become bound together through their experience and its interlocking states of aggression and fear. (There is always a 'third party' in this action in the form of a discarnate spirit who initiates the expression of violence, but *it* is not bound to the action or to the other two people in the same way.) This kind of 'imprisonment' of two people to each other and to the experience can persist beyond the physical life of either one or both of them, after which an even greater effort of consciousness and will is needed to free them.

It is not only experiences of violence that produce states of negative attachment. Frustration arising from real or imagined injustice can become the main focal point in a person's life; jealousy, envy, or hatred can be directed so strongly towards someone (who may have evoked it unwittingly), that it structures the entire mental world which the person in-breathes and within which he lives. A negative polarisation of this kind may so absorb the attention and energy of a person throughout his lifetime, that he in a sense *becomes* his frustration, his depression, or his jealousy. And when he passes out of physical life, he 'awakens' on an etheric plane in the same state. (In fact, what was a *mental* state on the physical plane becomes the person's *environment* in the etheric sphere.) Often, he does not even know that he has passed on to another plane of existence.

Every negative state of mind, indulged and inhabited on the physical plane, remains with the person during his etheric existence as part of his own nature as well as his environment. Change can only take place through his own will – and this may mean after long periods of time, when he becomes aware of the structure of this state and seeks for help to change it. Then the ones who are able to help can begin to teach him. With new knowledge, and through his own efforts, the person can dissolve this state and become free in time.

The 'rescue work' of freeing people from every degree of negative mental state is undertaken by millions of spirits on different levels, all of whom have gone through similar experiences in the course of their own evolution. A number of people in physical bodies are also engaged in rescue work. They provide a focus for *peace* and healing and give knowledge which those in spirit could not receive in any other way, often because they imagine they are still on a physical plane of existence and do not recognise forms of help offered by the spirit world. (In fact, many spirits find it impossible for a long time to accept that they have passed through the experience called 'death' and entered upon another plane of existence.) Rescue work is a gigantic task, the dimensions of which can scarcely be over-estimated.

Man's lack of awareness of his own being and his own motives and his failure to accept even existing knowledge about the inter-penetration of spirit and earth planes – the fact that all men are etheric beings NOW – makes him especially vulnerable. What he cannot see, and won't even accept the existence of, will continue to influence or use him until he desires a change in his own state of consciousness. The only real protection for the individual person against distortion from such inter-penetration by the spirit world is the light of his own consciousness.

The individual person exposes himself to danger through his own free will, whether consciously or unconsciously; his only protection lies in a different kind of use of his free will to procure understanding, to practise awareness, and to assume conscious responsibility for his life and its expression. This cannot be achieved in a moment, but protection commences with the realisation that every expression of a man's being has a vibration which is linked with other vibrations of the same quality in the unseen world around him. All expressions of impatience, anger, envy, bitterness, dissatisfaction, despair are vibrations of a certain kind which both excite and attract similar vibrations; expressions of sympathy, contentment, patience tune in to and attract their own quality of vibration in the universe. From moment to moment in the daily life of every person, through thoughts and actions, he can express and tune in to either positive or negative vibrations. If he desires protection against the influence of discarnate spirits who seek the expression of their own self wills through other human beings, he has firstly to guard against expresssing through *himself* the kind of vibration he does not want to attract. From moment to moment the choice is his own. It is as simple as that, requiring neither special teaching nor rituals; it is a choice – an exercise – open to everyone, according to his ability.

VI

When a person's awareness of his *kundalini sense*, and, through it, of the reality of his own etheric being, has grown and reached the point where it can begin to influence his self will and his willing, then a 'new' will is formed which can become a regenerating force for all his centres. Not only does a more efficient working of these centres become possible, but the quality of their working is altered; they work more harmoniously together, each one performing its own task.

This spiritual quickening becomes apparent first of all in the Sex Centre – which has not to do with physical sex but with the basis of a man's identity while in a physical body. Fantasy no longer dominates the working of this Centre, for the person's feeling of I-ness – his identity – no longer rests on imagination to the same extent. He is now re-connected with his own etheric being and intimations of knowledge and experience which are truly his own inner reality. Because he is not scattered in the way he used to be, his energy is more concentrated and available for use in new directions determined from within, by his 'new' will. Energy wells up and flows, often seeming inexhaustible in its supply.

The effect of a person's newly-awakened awareness of his own etheric reality on the Centre of Elimination can be to cleanse and heal the whole of his physical body. The internal organs may be strengthened, becoming more capable of dealing with the body's toxins, and the blood-stream cleared of impurities. This process may take a long time, but real and lasting health can only take place at all when the new will has been formed in the individual and when the imaginary self is no longer in control, producing the old habitual stresses and tensions in the body. All real physical healing must be preceded by a spiritual transformation in the person's being, after which healing is possible, not only of damage caused by former tensions but also of organic and inherited weaknesses as well, as far as the nature of these weaknesses permits. The physical body of the person can be made capable of performing all the tasks which belong to the true nature of his life, of whose structure he is now becoming aware; he is then given both the energy and the strength to express the purpose of his physical life on earth, where formerly imagination about himself usurped his energy and distorted the purpose and pattern of this life.

The Centre of Digestion is the reception centre for all that enters into a man from the physical world, for all sense impressions, all air, all food for the body. Usually tensions caused by the self will affect this Centre and make it incapable of receiving all the foods necessary for the maintenance of the body – except for sense impressions, all of which are *registered* regardless of tensions, but not truly received and sent on to the appropriate organ or centre. For man's receptivity to these impressions is selective, in accordance with his sense of self or 'I'. These tensions also reflect onto the physical organs to which the various foods and impressions are directed and which deal with their physical digestion, that is, the brain, lungs, stomach, pancreas, nervous systems, etc. The effect of the new will on this Centre is to relax tension generally and facilitate the digestion of all foods, the impressions being directed along their right channels to the nerve receptors and appropriate parts of the brain. In this way the real intelligence of the person may be increased, for intelligence can be equated with sensitivity to and awareness of the world in which he lives.

The Solar Plexus is a 'reception centre' or focus for all the etheric forces and vibrations with which a person is surrounded. Every human being – indeed, all life – is etheric now. He lives not only in the visible physical world but equally and more truly in the invisible one. It is through this invisible Centre, the Solar Plexus, and its reflection onto his physical spine that a man's contact with the etheric world occurs and is maintained; it is through this Centre that the etheric world contacts him.

The etheric world contains seven distinct stages or levels through which all men must evolve (and seven related forms or 'worlds' of distortion). These stages are composed of different qualities of experience and human expression; they reflect different forms of life. The seven stages represent *discrete* levels of experience which, taken together, contain every conceivable plane of etheric existence. The seven stages of evolution comprise co-existing, although separate, worlds of ever-increasing light and spirituality; whereas the worlds of distortion express types of spiritual malformation and levels of darkness. A man's etheric body interpenetrates his physical body, and so also do all the various etheric levels of vibration interpenetrate the physical plane of existence. The etheric is not 'other' or separate from the physical material world visible to man's physical sight. Any one of these distinct etheric levels can find expression on the physical plane; for men at all stages of evolution, and with every form of distortion, incarnate in physical bodies; and any spiritual level, from deepest darkness to greatest light, can be experienced by man while he is in a physical body, undergoing an expression of physical life on earth.

The Solar Plexus in a person is the door by which etheric vibrations enter his physical body. Just as the Centre of Digestion provides a door for the entrance of all sense impressions, and registers them with mechanical accuracy, so does the Solar Plexus provide an entrance for all etheric vibrations and record them with equal accuracy. All levels of vibration can enter a person through his Solar Plexus, although he may be completely unconscious of them or aware only of their physical effect upon him. Vibrations from the seven dark or lower etheric spheres enter and sometimes 'attack' a person through his Solar Plexus. So long as the person retains conscious control of and responsibility for his own mind, these lower vibrations can only gain entrance to his *body* through the Solar Plexus and affect his body alone, not his mind or his actions. If the person, for one reason or another, abdicates responsibility for his own mind and the actions that spring from it, then direct entry can be gained by any discarnate spirit that seeks its own expression through the medium of another person's body. A man may consciously relinquish sole control over his own mind and actions, which is his responsibility alone, or he may unconsciously relinquish it through motives whose true nature is hidden from himself; the results are similar, however, for he has opened himself to possession and all the dangers attendant thereon.

The other rôle of the Solar Plexus, apart from it being the door for the entry of etheric vibrations (some of which, like the Creative or Healing Force, are essential for maintaining man's physical life and without which his body would decay and die), has to do with its *conscious* use. This may best be explained in relation to the symbol of the wheel. The word *chakra* means a wheel. The *wheel* of the Solar Plexus, when consciously 'turned' by the person's will, can draw in a specific substance or vibration and then radiate it out again as directed by that person's consciousness. In this way the forces of Healing or Protection or the substance of *peace* can be consciously selected out of the etheric atmosphere surrounding a person, drawn in, and used by that person for himself or other people or for some form of animal or plant life. Once the wheel of the Solar Plexus is set in motion by the person's conscious will to draw in and re-direct a certain force or substance, it will continue to turn of its own accord, without further conscious direction, until the exercise is completed. (That is, for a period of five minutes. It is more effective, however, if the person continues to give the exercise his conscious attention.) The Solar Plexus cannot be used as a wheel in the person's unconscious states or before he has re-connected with his own etheric being through the *Kundalini* sense.

The re-connection of a man with his own etheric being affects the Solar Plexus by strengthening the nerves of which it is physically composed. Strengthening the nerves has the two-fold effect of making them both more resilient and more sensitive. Increase in sensitivity means an increase in the ability of the Solar Plexus to pick up etheric vibrations, whereas greater resilience means a certain amount of protection against intrusion by the lower etheric vibrations. The 'new' will implies a change in consciousness, an increase in the man's awareness of himself, and makes possible the working of the Solar Plexus as a wheel, so that new or additional forces can enter the person's body from outside, through the Solar Plexus – whether they are the Creative or Healing Force, the Force of Protection, or the *peace* substance.

Through the Solar Plexus a man tunes in to the whole of the

earth's etheric. This etheric includes all possible 'psychologies' of man, all possible states of mind which mankind can express. The *understanding* of these states, psychological or mental, does not come through the Solar Plexus because that Centre does not provide a framework or terms of reference in relation to which understanding arises. The *facts alone* are received and experienced (although only in part) through the Solar Plexus: in this way the seeds of understanding are sown; but they only grow through the inspiration, intuition, and knowledge that come through a man's Head Centre.

When a man re-connects with his own etheric being and the knowledge inherent in it, the effect is most apparent in relation to his Head Centre. The Head Centre is a focus or instrument which both receives vibrations of intuition and knowledge and sends them on to the man's own physical mind. When his physical mind reaches the stage of becoming truly receptive to this knowledge, so the Head Centre becomes increasingly sensitive in both its capacities. It becomes more receptive and more efficient as a transmitter of inspiration from the person's own etheric body, which inspiration consists largely of knowledge accumulated through previous experience the person has had on other planes of existence. And it also becomes more sensitive to the vibrations of guidance or help from other spiritual beings who are on the same positive wave length as the man himself and who draw near to offer assistance or advice from time to time, and at crucial moments in his life.

The new will, developed out of a person's re-connection with his own etheric being, also affects his Throat Centre. Its effect physically is to strengthen the organs associated with communication – the central nervous system and the thyroid and parathyroid glands. The desire to communicate is also strengthened. The desire to communicate comes, first of all, from the man's etheric being and this desire makes itself felt to greater effect. But as *desire* is only fully capable of expression when it is *willed*, so the new will in a man brings a new capacity for communication. The desire to communicate is not general or theoretical; it is related to specific changes in the man's being, in particular to the actual stage of his being and the form in which it is capable of expressing. It is also related to the person's renewed contact with his own inner source of inspiration and knowledge. The desire to communicate becomes, in part, the desire to communicate the inspiration which he himself receives and to share with others, in one way or another, the knowledge and understanding which he is discovering are the treasures of his own many experiences and 'lifetimes'. This new desire to communicate is, in a sense, a transformation of all former desires for self expression; only it is no longer a desire to express or glorify the imaginary self but rather the desire of a man to share with others the fruits – the truth – of his own experience. The ability to communicate by voice and word, and in every other way, is increased by this new will in a man.

The Heart Centre begins to develop only after a man has begun to reconnect with his own etheric being. Until that time comes, its potentialities are only latent. The Head and Throat Centres are at work in all men whatever stage of development they have reached. Everyone receives inspiration from his own etheric body and knowledge derived from his own previous experiences even though he often cannot connect with their vibrations, much less understand their origin. In every man there is a desire to communicate with the world around him, whatever form this may take. But the Heart Centre only begins to function after a person has reached a certain level of development where he no longer desires the experience, the expression, or the communication for himself. As long as his centre of gravity or feeling of identity is wholly in the Sex Centre, so long do his thoughts and actions serve and feed the physical self; only when the foundation of his identity has moved inwards, towards his own etheric reality, and he has begun to know who he is, does he become free to care about and learn who other people are. Until that time comes, other people – the world around him – do not exist for him as beings in their own right, apart from their role in relation to his own sense of identity.

The Heart Centre is the means by which a man can enter into and understand the nature of other beings separate from, but not *separated* from, himself. These may be other human beings or animals or various forms of plant life. Through the Heart Centre a person can connect with and learn to understand the nature of all life.

The word *empathy*, derived from Greek, best describes the working of the Heart Centre at this stage,[53] for it means consciously entering into the experience of another being. Through his Heart Centre a man receives the vibrations or impulses from another being which provide him with the facts about that being's nature, present state, and inner meaning – or *signature* (as Jakob Boehme described it). These facts are actually *experienced* by the man through his Heart Centre; it is this experience from which his knowledge about and understanding of the other being derive. This is the beginning of what may be called *objective experience*, which is the direct experience of facts or qualities uninfluenced by the personal mind of the experiencer. From this seed-experience can grow the ability to experience and, through experience, understand many aspects and levels of reality.

The Centre of Digestion in a man receives impressions from the physical world around him: all food, air, and sense impressions. They are registered automatically. The Solar Plexus in a man receives impressions from the etheric world in the same way. Both centres can work in half-light or even in darkness; neither depends for its working on a man's awareness of himself. The Heart Centre, on the contrary, does not work automatically at all and is only called into operation by the extension of a man's consciousness. This does not come about through any abstract desire for knowledge or in order to satisfy some intellectual curiosity. A man's *conscious willing* can only proceed from a desire to go out to, or give to, another being. Then only does the Heart Centre – in response to the man's own desire, consciousness, willing – begin to function and pick up vibrations from the total reality of the particular person or being, at a particular moment in time. It picks up physical vibrations – which the Centre of Digestion may also have registered: it picks up etheric vibrations – which may also have been received by the Solar Plexus. It also picks up vibrations from the inner nature of the other being and, most important of all, receives *all* the separate vibrations as a single experience of the whole person or being, in which each impression is related to the whole pattern. Every impression is registered by the Heart Centre, but coordination takes place through the *experience*. This experience is only possible through the Heart Centre. The Heart Centre is the focal point through which all experience of *objective reality* is possible. The objective reality of a human being reveals where that person is in terms of his own spiritual evolution; or, if it refers to an animal or plant which does not evolve spiritually, the pattern of objective reality reflects the perfect etheric form of the particular animal or plant.

Objective reality also reveals what a person or animal or plant needs at a particular moment in time. Through his Heart Centre alone a man can have an objective experience of the other person's (or object's) physical or spiritual needs, undistorted by the partial knowledge given by his other centres and uncoloured by his own fantasies. Through his Heart Centre he can know his own responsibility in relation to each person or being and what action (if any) he must take himself from moment to moment.

It is the 'new' will in a man which makes possible the working and the development of his Heart Centre. Through re-connecting with his own etheric being, and the growth of this new will, he becomes able for the first time to experience objective reality: to perceive and experience things *as they are* in himself and in the world around him. This ability does not arise overnight but grows very slowly. The commencement of this ability to experience objective reality, however, marks an entirely new stage in the man's own spiritual evolution: it is one of the few truly discrete steps in the whole pattern of his spiritual growth. Its growth continues throughout the eternity of the man, because there is no limit to objective reality and no limit to the new levels and aspects of it which man can experience.

The new will in a man makes possible not only the *experience* of objective reality through his Heart Centre but also the will to act responsibly in relation to this experience. This means to act in relation to what is revealed to him from moment to moment, allowing his actions to remain flexible and proceed from his ever-changing, ever new experience of what IS. It means acting (or not acting) in relation to the total need of the other person or being, in terms of the greatest good for his spiritual purpose or meaning. Until there is this 'new' will a person would be unable to act purely from his perception of another man's needs; all his actions would be influenced by his own attitudes, desires, or fantasies. Thus the new will makes it possible for a man to begin to express and carry out one of the most important purposes inherent in his own spiritual nature, which is to aid the growth and regeneration of the world around him.

ADDENDUM

Man – not plant or animal life – was the original 'creation'. All men were created simultaneously. A few evolved spiritually but the vast majority did not evolve or evolved very little. The ones who did evolve were concerned with the state of other men and, discovering the capacity in themselves for creation, created other forms of life as *forms* only for men to enter into and gain varieties of experience through and provide what they hoped would be an impetus to man's further development. These forms were plant and animal forms similar to (but not identical with) those which exist today, only they did not then have independent existence as separate species but existed *solely* as forms for the experience of human beings on the etheric planes. This was the first creation undertaken by spiritual beings – that is, by more highly-evolved men – to help the rest of mankind evolve spiritually. The creation of plant and animal forms as *separate* species, with independent existence, was a much later creation, undertaken by individual persons who had themselves evolved through the different forms. They created the separate species out of gratitude for their own experiences and because they had come to love the forms. (The *physical* creation of these species was yet another and very much later creation, which was part of the creation of the physical earth, undertaken for the same reasons as the original creation of the plant and animal forms, namely, to provide an impetus for the evolution of individual men, as well as to remind them of their experiences within these forms.)

From the middle of the nineteenth century onwards the nature of physical life on earth had so changed that there was need for a much higher degree of spiritual evolution before the individual person could benefit from his incarnation. If someone were born on earth today in a more primitive (that is, undeveloped but not distorted) etheric state, he simply could not benefit from his experience in the complex, machine and material – oriented social structures which exist everywhere. His spiritual being could become distorted and his own spiritual evolution set back for a long period of time.

For the past hundred years and more the earth has become increasingly peopled with persons who have arrived 'before their time', that is, been born before they were sufficiently advanced spiritually for the experience of an earth-life to be of value for them. By the last quarter of the twentieth century, seventy per cent of the people on earth had taken on physical lives before they were sufficiently evolved for their lives to be spiritually fruitful. Moreover, through a preponderance of spiritually under-developed people on earth, the conditions of life under which *all* people had to live had deteriorated so much by that time that it was difficult for anyone to find his own individual expression through normal physical life, and a natural form of growth for his etheric being was impossible. Social structures had become more gross and all-encompassing and, by stressing the collective grouping rather than individual expression, made it increasingly difficult for any person to stand out against collective pressures, to take individual decisions and personal initiative, and to become truly accessible to the voice of his own conscience. The quality of life – which resides wholly in the ability of individuals to express individually – declined and is continuing to decline throughout the whole of the twentieth century.

This lack of spiritual development in the majority of people on earth may be defined as an insufficient development of the three upper *chakras* through which a person's etheric, or spiritual, body expresses. One of these centres might be more highly developed in some people, but usually all three centres are under-developed and the etheric beings of these people express solely through the three lower centres. The evolutionary stage has not yet been reached where there is either the necessity or the possibility for a sense of purpose, direction, or guidance. In all these people the preponderance of development lies with the *chakras* belonging to the physical body, through which the physical or animal nature expresses. This represents the stage of expression natural for their etheric beings. If they had remained in the etheric sphere, instead of incarnating, their evolution would have proceeded gradually and naturally; but by their precipitate entrance into physical bodies, they run the risk of prolonging this stage and making their evolution beyond it much more difficult. For their etheric beings are wholly caught up in a material-physical orientation that structures and even ensnares their minds far beyond the natural limitations of the physical life. Furthermore, a preponderance of such spiritually under-developed people on earth influences the structuring of *all* human societies to the detriment of those people who are more evolved spiritually and who need a more differentiated social environment and culture for their beings to express through and grow.

The majority of people who are 'born before their time' enter an earth experience because of their dependence upon other persons who have taken on, or are about to take on, a physical life. They may also be drawn into physical life through some vibration of excitement which attracts them. But it is always their dependence upon – or their identification with – another person which is the primary cause of their will to be born into an earth-body. (The 'other person' may or may not have been born before his or her time. If he or she is born with sufficient spiritual preparation – that is, at the 'right time' for him – the physical life-experience will proceed naturally and not be adversely affected by the subsequent birth of someone who is so closely dependent upon him.) It is not impossible for a person who has been born before his time to develop spiritually, but it depends upon the strength of his own will and the stage of its evolution, for great efforts have to be made to do so. If there has not been sufficient development of will, the ability to make such effort does not exist.

A person may also have a will which is one-sided in its strength and direction or closely identified with the will of the person through whom he was attracted into a physical life in the first place. A strong and rigid self will is evidence of obsession or possession – or sometimes both. More than a third of the people who are born before their time have strong and rigid wills.

The strength of will which a person possesses in his physical life has always been developed through the effort needed to pursue a specific line of direction while still in the etheric spheres. A specialised or one-sided development in the person's being appears in the form of a 'talent' on the physical plane: a talent for some form of art, music, research, money-making, and so on. Whatever the talent, it represents a direction set *before* the entrance of that person into his physical life; his being was already centred upon this single expression or this one-sided development which his will procured – and in relation to which his will was vastly strengthened.

Some people, who nevertheless belong to this group of strong willed people, *appear* passive or 'weak' willed. Seeming passivity often hides obstinacy, and the will in this person may be strong in its resistance to other wills rather than in expressing its own. This kind of one-sidedness takes a negative form and attracts to itself various forms of frustration or depression, and usually possession by discarnate spirits whose expressions take the same form. In fact, even strong-willed people with a more positive form of expression can also exhibit a pronounced obstinacy and the accompanying negative forms of expression as well.

People with this kind of will always attract, at some point during the course of their physical lives, discarnate spirits with a similar one-sided development who add force or strength to their own wills. Such possession, even of a temporary nature – which it rarely is – makes a new evolution of will for that person almost impossible. His physical life is usually 'wasted' and he must await a return to an etheric plane of existence before his will can be extricated from the will of the discarnate spirit – or spirits – and from his own one-sided development, and begin anew the slow process of evolution.

In about half the cases of people with this kind of strong will, a more comprehensive form of spirit possession is expressed which, again, originated in experiences prior to the person's physical life on earth. These experiences – unresolved on the etheric plane – are carried with the person into his physical life and affect that life in the form of being possessed (from time to time) by the discarnate spirit to whom these previous experiences relate. Because the unresolved relationships are usually of a negative nature, so the form of possession is usually a negative one and hangs over the physical life of the person like a cloud, interfering with and often cutting him off from a natural expression of his life. The lives of eighteen per cent of the people on earth today may be described in this way. (It is important to realise that the personal attachments which draw these people into physical life in the first place are never identical with the possessions which hold them back and make impossible a natural and complete expression of that life. These 'attachments', representing the weak and under-developed side of the person, are always to members of the opposite sex; whereas the 'possessions' occur through the developing will and its experiences which one or both parties failed to work out or resolve before entering upon a physical life.)

Strong will and single-mindedness are often highly valued as attainments worthy of emulation by whole societies on earth, whereas in fact they represent as much a spiritual *weakness* as do any forms of so-called neurotic obsession. The apparent 'strength' is a kind of rigidity which will have to be broken down before any real growth in being can take place.

Slightly fewer than two-thirds of the people who have been born before their time – that is, forty-five per cent of all people on earth today – should not have been born at all because their beings are too undeveloped and primitive for them to make use of the opportunities for growth which life in a physical body presents. Their entrance into physical life, while made possible by a close relationship with someone already in or entering into a physical body, was motivated solely by a form of *greed*; without this motivation of greed, a physical life would never have been sought at this stage. While still living in the etheric spheres, these people were attracted by the baubles of material civilisation – the possessions and the activities which they saw people on earth enjoying, and it was these sights which fascinated and awoke in them a desire for physical life. This was not a desire for experience but only for material possessions and activities that would titilate the senses, for they as yet knew nothing about the spiritual growth which is possible for every human being. They came into physical bodies solely to enjoy: there is no other purpose for their life on earth; they have completely forgotten their previous existence and the etheric sphere in which their beings have true reality.

Only thirty per cent of all people on earth at this time, in the last quarter of the twentieth century, are capable of profitting from their experience in physical bodies; for them alone is *experience* in itself of primary importance, and the wisdom or understanding which can be learned from such experience. Among the first group of people with strong wills, there are those who *know about* spiritual growth and the purpose of spiritual life – but are unable to act from that knowledge during their lifetimes. It is only people in this last group – that is, people who have incarnated at the *right time for them* – who are capable of real growth and development during their physical lives. They alone have the potentiality for taking on added responsibilities for other people and creating conditions within which not only the flowering of men's physical natures becomes possible but also opportunities exist to learn about the true nature of man and his potentiality for spiritual growth. They alone can give society the structures men need for their spiritual evolution.

[1]Whether aleopathy, homeopathy, naturopathy, spiritual healing, or other.

[2]The quality of the healing power is always directly related to the level of being of the healer and of the spirit being whom he attracts.

[3]There is a source of healing which transcends the creative forces and is used by persons who have evolved beyond the etheric sphere altogether; but a discussion of this does not belong to the teaching about *pranayama* and healing by the pranic forces.

[4]There is no *absolute* protection on the physical earth although there is in all other spheres. Absolutes do not exist at all on earth and all 'certainties', whatever their nature, are what might be called 'ninety percent certain'. There is always the possibility of failure because of the nature of the physical creation which is separate from – although linked with – the etheric creation and has a momentum of its own. So it is with the substance of *protection*.

[5]It does not exist on the etheric planes or in the etheric sphere except as part of man's intrinsic nature. It does not exist in plant or animal life on the etheric spheres – but only in man.

[6]This was particularly true in earlier times when the species were in process of physical formation, although it is still true to a lesser extent.

[7]With occasional exceptions in a number of vertebrates, where the odd animal

individuates and becomes capable of separate and individual responses and relationships.

[8]This 'materialisation' of every expression of life in the etheric sphere, in denser forms, was not originally envisaged but came about at a very much later stage as a way of dealing with the problems of spiritual entropy, in an attempt to give new impetus to the evolution of individual human beings.

[9]The creation of physical forms, on the physical earth, was from simple to increasingly complex and worked *in reverse* to the original etheric creation, where man was created first, *before* any other etheric forms of plant or animal life were created.

[10]The history of Organic Life on earth *appears* 'evolutionary' in retrospect and unrelated to the working of real and prior spiritual creation on the etheric plane.

[11]There were two separate and distinct acts of creation which proceeded from different starting points and involved different kinds of process. On the etheric plane, man was created first and *all* plant and animal species were created much 'later' as *separate* manifestations and not as part of any evolutionary or inter-species growth process. The creation of the physical earth was very much 'later' still and manifested slowly within a 'time' scale and through evolutionary progression from simple to complex forms. Here, the *physical* form of man was evolved last of all, and etheric beings only began to enter into physical bodies for an experience of life on a physical earth after long ages of 'time' – after the evolutionary process had reached the stage of preparing adequate physical bodies for him to inhabit.

[12]The individual physical animal is always a new creation without prior etheric existence. *Separate* spiritual identity did not exist at all on etheric planes prior to the physical manifestation of mammal life.

[13]There have been many physical forms into which individual men have incarnated, commencing with the earliest forms of proto-man. These forms represent more primitive stages in man's etheric or spiritual evolution. Man never incarnated in the physical forms of plant or animal life. As men evolved spiritually, so the physical forms of mankind progressed as vehicles for his physical manifestation.

[14]See Addendum at the conclusion of this section, p.136ff.

[15]The etheric *body* of Organic Life, which is a whole and distinct etheric body, was created after the physical earth was first created but *before* any physical forms of plant or animal life were created. Before the physical earth was created there was no such body of Organic Life to which the separate, etheric plant and animal species belonged.

[16]For example, no animals were created to eat other animals. The carnivorous 'instinct', even of the predators, was not originally *natural* to them but came about as a reflection of man's behaviour and the vibrations emanating from man. The reaction of the cat family to anything that moves is of the same origin: the response of a highly sensitive animal nature to the emanations from man's mind and from his behaviour.

[17]The word is not proto-Sanskrit in origin – although it is of equally ancient derivation, nor was this knowledge about the *kundalini sense* taught in the original, Sumerian Yoga teaching. It was taken into that teaching in its early stages through contact with another culture.

[18]See Ernest Wood's book, *Yoga*, Pelican Books, 1959, and its references to 'Kundalini'.

[19]All the centres or *chakras* contain energy-reservoirs on which they draw for their functioning or use.

[20]It is not wholly this, because the physical sexual urge is a distinct and powerful urge in man, especially in the early years of maturity.

[21]There is a trait in the etheric beings of all people, until they reach a certain stage, that desires to hold on to or keep secret some bit of knowledge or some possession. This desire for secrecy is a manifestation of the desire for personal power.

[22]As the ancient 'schools' became more *exo*-teric and the Mysteries became popularised, so the external rites of initiation became rituals in which an increasing number of people participated, the criterion for participation being *faith* or adherence to doctrine and not knowledge – or *self*-knowledge and a supposed growth of being, as had originally been requirements for initiation. An aspect of this ritual which existed in many religious sects – most clearly formulated in the Eleusinian Mysteries – was the act of 'eating the God', literally or symbolically. Through this ancient act or ritual the person believed he acquired some of the attributes or power of the One he ate, or made contact with Him, or felt himself protected and secure in the meaning and definition of his life.

[23]This is not a description of any kind of state in which the person 'leaves his body', as some people imagine. It is *not* possible for any person to leave his physical body until the time comes for his passing. All such descriptions are either phantasies or relate to an experience of extended awareness of mind which is interpreted as 'leaving the body'.

[24]Symbolised by the apex of the triangle in the Diagram of Man or 'Enneagram'.

[25]These are not two separate creative forces but different manifestations of the universal Creative Force, one having the capacity for creation on the *physical* plane and the other – the Creative Imagination – being able to create anything, anywhere in the etheric or spiritual spheres.

[26]This is not 'merely' a mental world but the actual world in which each person has his existence, a world which is more truly 'real' for him than the material-physical objects which he takes as real. For it is this world, which he himself created, which defines his relationship to all things and to all people.

[27]There are artists who think that they create directly on canvas, without idea or plan of more than the most shadowy form. They are either ignorant of the process of creation at work in themselves or else are unconscious *mediums*, whose hands and minds are used by another's will to create *his* art-form.

[28]Mozart is supposed to have heard the whole of his 40th Symphony in a single moment of time.

[29]The word 'meditation' is said to derive from the Latin *meditatio*, and there are various connotations of the word in most European languages which cover a wide range of meanings: to plan something, to give attention to one thing by a process of limitation or exclusion, absorption in an interior state to the exclusion of exterior phenomena, attentiveness, etc. To go further back, the word derives from a word meaning *to be in the middle*, and it is this which gives a clue to the true meaning of meditation, that is, to stand in the middle of life with interior and exterior awareness.

[30]*Effort* is expended in relation to the dream or fantasy – and often it is considerable effort, but this is not the same kind of effort as that required to seek the intrinsic reality in things.

[31]To act without the desire to alter something means acting in relation to the need of the particular situation, the needs of the other people involved; it is not the *re-action* of the self will.

[32]Although these essential conditions can be overlaid with much that does not *belong* to a person's life through the will of other people or the general conditions that exist on the earth at any particular time.

[33]Ideas or attitudes founded on an illusion of *equality* of people or 'talents', and the envy from which such ideas ultimately spring, only distract a person from what belongs to his own life. Whole societies, and now human life generally on earth, are distorted in their true function as a framework for individual human endeavour, by the predominance of a philosophy of human equality. Individual lives are distorted by the idea of 'rights' that belong to them and by the kinds of protection which technologically advanced societies provide against discovering in physical terms the

nature of their own strengths and weaknesses. In this way, most people are discouraged from accepting the reality of their own natures, which is the *only* starting point for spiritual growth and the sole reason for their earth lives.

[34]This is another form of the basic *pranayama* exercise described on pp.80-1.

[35]The two channels on either side of the spinal column exist *only* in man's invisible physical body and are, in fact, not two separate channels at all but one continuous and unbroken circular tube, extending from the Sex to the Head Centre and back. Only the third or central channel actually exists within the spinal column of the physical body of man.

[36]They do *not* develop the centres beyond the stage which the person had attained to spiritually before his entrance into a physical body, but only correct the maladjustments acquired in the process of that physical life.

[37]Any misappropriation of function by one or more centres, which existed *prior* to the person's entry into physical life, is *not* cured in this way. Nor is there any certainty that the malfunctioning acquired during the physical life can be completely cured through these exercises.

[38]Their development beyond this point or stage is another matter altogether.

[39]There are in fact twelve essential or *spiritual* types of human being which were created in the beginning and correspond to the twelve tones of the octave, each note or type representing a different quality of whole (not partial) vibration or eternal being. But the *reality* lies not in the note as such but in the individual human beings through which it is expressed. And it is the *individual* human expression which is eternal not any abstraction.

[40]This 'natural unity' may be a state of spiritual distortion or imbalance which belonged to the person *before* his entry into physical life but of which he is unaware because of all that life in a physical body has laid over it. It is the underlying state of his own etheric being of which he has to become aware.

[41]The 'natural unity' may already have been distorted at the time of his birth through prenatal experiences within his mother.

[42]Even if it is a *distorted* wholeness.

[43]He may re-experience certain aspects of, or connections from, his previous etheric existence without understanding what they are, and so attribute these experiences to another cause.

[44]Many forms of organised religious expression, Christian and non-Christian, are based on this desire in men. For example, the Pentecostal Movement derives much of its impetus from this factor in man and many of its dangers are explained in the text above.

[45]All forms of trance mediumship, whatever their purported aim – whether healing or guidance or other, are based on this kind of possession. And the spirit who enters into the physical being of another person, substituting his will with its own, is always from one of the lower spheres and to a certain extent distorted in its own being. No spirit from any of the higher etheric spheres would ever enter into such a relationship, because his own understanding of the nature and meaning of the individual will, and the conditions necessary for its growth, would make it impossible for him to do so.

[46]But these facts are taken out of context and distorted.

[47]Sometimes its use is unconscious, and in such a case its transmission may be compared with that of a dangerous disease through a carrier. But even if the agent is unconscious of the purpose and intent of the destructive substance he is transmitting, the person or persons using him are fully aware of what they are doing.

[48]See Addendum at the end of this chapter.

[49]The word, *religion*, relates to the Latin 'religare' or 'ligare', meaning to bind back, secure, hold fast.

[50]A rejection of atheistic system of belief, such as Marxism in its various forms,

labels the person as unbeliever, heretic, foolish, or, at worst, insane, but the person does not have his spiritual salvation or goals or growth-pattern challenged. This is because such systems deny the existence of any life other than the visible, material-physical one. This denial, of course, causes other – and, in some senses, worse – forms of mental distortion.

[51]This does not mean that every activity of a certain kind – e.g., all spirit healing – is the 'work of the Devil'. The nature of an activity depends upon the individual person's relationship to it.

[52]Activities do not have intrinsic natures. Their quality always depends upon the being of the person performing it and his motive.

[53]There are other stages and other expressions of the Heart Centre which belong to a much later point in man's evolution.

CHAPTER FOUR

PRATYAHARA

The fifth segment of the Yoga teaching, as it has been passed down over the ages in its purely oral form, is called *Pratyahara* and has to do with understanding the nature of mind, in particular the structure of mind which is comprised of all the senses and through which each person is in touch with the world in which he lives and moves. Through his own particular sense structure, his own mind, each person's world – the only world in which he lives – is created. The word, *Pratyahara*, means in fact this structure or sense organ[1] – this most important passive organ of man's mind, by which *everything* coming from outside the individual's own etheric body is received.[2] *All* etheric and physical data from the man's environment are received by this mental organ in himself; *what* is received and *how* it is received depend upon the nature and development of this mental sense organ. Its nature is a reflection of the man's level of being, of the stage of his mind-development. To this structure of *Pratyahara* belong the two centres, or *chakras*, in man which have to do with the reception of impressions, both physical and etheric, from outside,[3] that is, the Digestive Centre and the Solar Plexus. The Head Centre belongs only in part to the *Pratyahara*, insofar as it is the receiver of guidance or vibrations of help from the etheric world around a person. The Head Centre is primarily a focus for knowledge that comes from within the person's own etheric being and so belongs to another aspect of his mind altogether.

I

Mind is etheric in nature and is *in fact*, not merely symbolically, a microcosm of the whole etheric world in which all men live and have their being. Mind is a replica of the entire etheric universe of being known to man.

The mind of every person on earth may be thought of as *potentially* a seven-storey house, every level of which opens out into a different sphere of existence in the etheric world. It may also be thought of as a house having *fourteen* possible rooms which a person may inhabit. These fourteen compartments open out into the seven 'upper' etheric levels, through which each person will progress during the aeons of his spiritual evolution, and into the seven 'lower' etheric spheres or forms of life into which men can descend and where they express their inner states of distortion or perversion. Man's mind consists of fourteen kinds of mental *state* which open out onto fourteen kinds of *place*; these vary from the deepest form of darkness and most negative or perverted states of being to one where light and truth are most perfectly reflected. The place of greatest darkness exists for a man when all light and truth have been rejected by his own will; in fact, were it not for the 'darkness' of a man's state of mind – of the states of mind of many people – such a place could not exist, for the *place* of darkness in the etheric sphere has been created by those people who have willed darkness rather than light and have created, first of all for themselves, mental states into which no light or truth could enter. As a *state of mind* reflects outwards and creates *place* so a person becomes enclosed in a world of his own making. On the highest level a man's mind will reflect all that exists in the etheric universe; for a man to reach this level, he must will to know and experience all things as they are. And so, in this same way, all gradations of darkness and light are created by a man's will and experienced both as state of mind and place.

Every man, whatever the stage of his being, has a mind which contains all fourteen possible states and opens out onto the fourteen etheric levels or places. When a man passes out of his physical body he still possesses the same mind. Even at the seventh level of light, where the mind of a man is wholly cleansed and free of all divisions, it will still be a microcosm of the etheric universe for it will accurately reflect every level of darkness and light. And through his mind the person will then be able to perceive the whole Etheric and know the details of its meaning and structure. It will not reflect in the way any other mind reflects, for every mind is unique because it has been created by the person's own unique experiences. Only when that person goes beyond the Etheric altogether does his mind cease to reflect the etheric levels because he is outside their orbit; but when he re-enters the etheric spheres, his mind again reflects their entire structure in accordance with its own nature. A man cannot escape the nature of mind; he cannot alter the fact that it is, in a sense, related to everything in the etheric universe. He is, through his mind, indirectly connected with every level of despair and darkness and perversion – and, equally, with every level of hope and light and intelligence – in the universe. Even at the seventh level, when a man has gone through all the etheric experiences that belong to his own being and transmuted them, he is still connected with every etheric level and is, to a degree, responsible for all that exists in this universe. Until the whole of mankind is redeemed and regenerated, so long will all men remain part of and responsible for one another and all that exists in the etheric world.[4]

All worlds were created by Mind and are continuing to be created by Mind. *State* exists before *place*. *All* creation is through individual minds and there has been no creation apart from this. No abstract or impersonal forces ever created rock or plant or animal – let alone man. Nothing[5] existed before individual mind, that is the minds of individual men.

Through long aeons of evolution, individual minds have created innumerable places of existence, first etheric and then physical, and structured and furnished them with inanimate and animate forms. Without knowledge of the laws of Creation to begin with, and unconscious of himself and the nature of the Etheric Substance, man created a whole universe through his own mind. Only at later stages in his evolution, did man begin to become conscious of himself and of the nature of the Etheric and so begin more consciously to explore and create. As individual men evolved, the nature of their states altered and, out of these altered states, they created new *habitations*. Others who followed after these 'explorers' entered into the places or habitations already created for them. Every stage of evolution towards the light, every manifestation on the path of growth, is created by individual men who are truly explorers and trail-breakers. Likewise, all manifestations of perversion and distortion which exist in the universe are created by individual men. There is nothing in the etheric universe or beyond, no aspect of objective reality: no place or structure of place or denizen of place, which has not been created by individual men and women.

The mind of the individual person is not merely circumscribed and defined by its particular physical expression, in its limited physical body, but partakes of the whole extension of Mind. This means not only *spatial* extension – an extension into every possible place and state, but participation in the creative potentiality of Mind as well. The mind of every individual human being contains the ability to create, for good or ill. And every man, whether consciously or unconsciously, makes use of this ability.

Through their Creative Imaginations men create the worlds in which they live – or adapt and select from and work upon the world into which they have been born. All this proceeds unconsciously. Each person's mind, unconsciously and in accordance with its own nature, creates a 'self' and a world for it to inhabit; this becomes 'the world' through which that person apprehends and experiences every form of life around him. This creation of his own mind is his own *subjective reality* – not less real for its 'subjectivity' than any other form of reality. This is what he takes as real and experiences as real. But however real it is for him, it is not real for other people; for *subjective* reality is not the same as *objective* reality.

Man's mind is also capable of creating not only those forms of reality which are true for him, but *objective reality* as well. The creation of all forms of objective reality is a result of the combined effort of Creative Imagination and Will. When a person's individual will – the sum of all his separate wills – enters into the act of creation, whatever the direction or form of its expression, the result is one of objective reality. For a man to will what his mind has created there must be a certain degree of consciousness. Every kind of objective reality, every manifestation which has reality for other people as well as for the man who created it, is the result of his will and his consciousness. Subjective reality, which is only real for the individual person, is primarily the result of his Creative

Imagination;[6] for this *subjective* reality to become *objective* it has to be acted upon by his will and consciousness.

Both kinds of reality exist at every human level. At every level men and women live and experience through their own forms of subjective reality. Slowly, these forms of reality change or are altered as the individual learns, grows, and evolves. Also, at every level in the long process of human evolution, there have been individuals in whom will has evolved more quickly and who have used their wills to create new environments for other people to dwell in as well as themselves. All the levels through which human beings evolve towards the light have been created in this way by individual persons, inspired by their Creative Imaginations, wills, and consciousness. This process of creation is still going on as men continue to evolve beyond the already-known states and experiences and places.

But men do not only create *positive* environments or forms of expression for others to experience; they can also create distortions, demons, and places of darkness for people to inhabit. The process of *negative* creation is exactly the same as it is for a positive expression: it depends upon active *willing* and upon a certain degree of consciousness on the part of the individual.

People can spend part – even a large part – of their lives dwelling in a distorted or negative environment of their own creation; so long as it is their own subjective reality it does not directly affect other people. They are also in some measure, at some point in their physical lives – or later on – in an etheric existence, open to a form of help which can free them and make possible new expressions of growth. If, however, a person actively wills his own form of distorted reality he can create out of it a reality with *objective* existence which envelops everyone involved with that person in some degree of the same distortion. That person's 'reality' has not only been projected outside himself but actively *created* and given independent existence according to its inherent nature. The *de-creation* of this form of reality is much more complex and takes much longer to accomplish, for it is not only the mind of a single individual which is involved, but the minds of many individuals and a *set of facts which has developed a life of its own*.

The vast majority of men in physical bodies live out their lives in only one storey of the multi-storey structure of the etheric world, in one very small part of their total mind potential. In fact, most men take many many 'lifetimes' of etheric experience on one level before they progress onto a higher level in their individual pattern of evolution. A few people are able to pass through many experiences and several etheric levels during a physical lifetime; this was the original intention or aim with regard to life in a physical body, but it is no longer usual. Most men spend their whole lives not only in one storey in the etheric – or mental – universe, but live in a very small segment of that storey. The segment in which they live constitutes what is *real* for them. The dimensions of their own personal reality remain relatively unchanged throughout their lives until they begin to realise that what they take for reality has, in fact, been created by themselves. Only then does the nature of their experience begin to change as their conception of reality becomes less rigid. When they begin to see that the mental forms which structure their thinking, seeing, and therefore their lives are products of their own imagination or the imagination of the society in which they live, so they begin to become loosened from that conception of reality which they have hitherto taken for granted.

Reality is never fixed or constant but always relative to the person and time. What is *real* for someone at one time, and in one state or on one level of being, becomes *unreal* at another. What one person takes as real and acts from as real, is *real for him.* It is in the nature of the *kind of reality* created by men at a certain level of existence that this fact of relativity is not understood, for at this level the forms of man's thinking are dualistic and absolute; absolutes are axiomatic to his thinking, definitions are rigid. At times of cultural fissiparation and when particular social cohesions begin to break down,[7] the 'absolutes' or axioms on which these cultures and their thinking/behaviour patterns were based are thrown into question; the thinking of the men living in these societies may become temporarily less rigid but is often confused. True relativity of thinking does not result from such cultural or social changes; individual men and women only learn to think relatively through growth in their own personal states of awareness.

Reality is all that people *take as real* with their minds at a certain level. Regardless of the state of any particular culture or society, at any one time, it may contain individuals from any or all of the seven levels of being and with any of the seven possible forms of distortion. All these levels and forms can co-exist in the same physical society at any one time and each level or form will open out onto a different conception and experience of reality.

For every human being in any given society, there are three out of the many possible etheric levels or mental states which can be more or less real for him during his lifetime. The first of these is the mental or etheric stage which he inhabits most of the time, and the small segment or expression of it peculiar to himself. The second one is the negative counterpart, of distortion or perversion, to the positive stage he should naturally inhabit. This is the state into which he can fall or touch momentarily through his own wilfulness, strong emotion, self-imagination, desire for power – or which he can come to inhabit entirely. The third state which it is possible for him to experience is the one above his ordinary level which he can also touch occasionally and even unexpectedly. This is not necessarily another *level* of being, but may be a higher manifestation of the level he ordinarily inhabits.[8] A person is not only able to touch or momentarily experience one or more stages other than the one he normally inhabits, he can also begin to *inhabit* either a higher or lower level of mind. Movement of being, either upwards or downwards, is not only possible for everyone, it is implicit in all human life. Such movement is even implicit in the smallest choices a person makes throughout his physical lifetime. Even where change in the level of being a person inhabits is not obvious, it nonetheless takes place in everyone, and the direction in which a man's choices tend will indicate the changes in his being. There is no such thing as a stable or static mental state for a man; there must be movement, and the direction of this movement is either upwards, towards the level above – even if its actual achievement may be many lifetimes away – or downwards towards a lower level, which is a level of distortion and abnormality.[9]

Mind is etheric in nature; the Etheric Spheres can equally well be thought of as having a mental or psychological nature. The terms are interchangeable; even more important, the substances of Mind and Etheric are essentially the same substance. There is only *one* etheric substance.

Etheric Substance consists of one primary substance which has the possibility of limitless forms. These forms are created by the Creative Force which is, itself, part of the Etheric Substance. In other words, the Creative Force is not separate from the Etheric Substance, being the more active aspect of its nature. For the Etheric Substance combines both active and passive functions; it 'creates', and at the same time contains within itself all possible materials for the work of creation, and it is also the crucible within which the act of creation takes place.

But the Creative Force does not activate itself; it does not call itself into action or contain its own aims, motives, or direction. It is an *agent* that can only be called into action by *will*, that is, the individual will of a man. The activity of the Creative Force is always under the authority of an individual will (whether the person is in a physical or an etheric body makes no difference) from which derives aim, motive, and direction for the particular creation. All *etheric* forms of Organic Life, both plant and animal (excluding man), were called into being by this process of creation, prior to their physical manifestation. And the wills of individual men have initiated the physical creation of every living form on earth. For out of the etheric forms of plant and animal life physical manifestation does not *automatically* proceed without a new action of will. *All* creation – each new creation – starts with the will to create in which aim or purpose is embodied. This aim is impressed upon the Creative Force which then begins to act from it, on and within the Etheric Substance, selecting and developing the materials necessary for the creation of the particular form in which the aim will be embodied. This process of creation is the same in both the etheric and physical spheres; but in the physical sphere the Creative Force also continues to work within each form to maintain, repair, and heal it during the limited duration of its existence.

Mind is composed of Etheric Substance and contains all possible forms. But Mind does not create its own forms; it is, like all Etheric

Substance, the material out of which all mental forms are created by man's faculty of imagination – which is the active aspect of Mind. The process of creation is the same in Mind as it is in the Etheric Substance. The Creative Imagination in a man is the mental counterpart of the Creative Force within the Etheric Substance; it is activated by man's will – or self will – through the medium of an aim, purpose, or motive held by that will. It is through his own mind that the aims or underlying motives of a man are given form and made real to himself.

The Creative Imagination in a man is not equal in creative power to the Creative Force because it derives from it. It has the capacity to create only what is *real for itself*, not what is real for anyone else. The Creative Imagination in a man possesses *in itself* only the ability to create subjective reality. Most of what it creates is unconscious or, at best, semi-conscious to the person, for the will which activates the Creative Imagination is dispersed, diffuse, and acts through many and unconscious motives. Where the will of a man is working with a higher degree of consciousness there can be a *second* act of creation which turns the subjective reality into objective reality. This is discussed in another place.

What is important here is the realisation that each man possesses the ability to create – and does create – his own mental world which he alone inhabits and which constitutes reality for him. The 'gods' or 'demons' he creates for himself, out of his own *mind-stuff*, have as great a validity for him as do the physical manifestations of Organic Life in the world about him. This fact can scarcely be over-emphasised: that each man inhabits a world which he has created for himself – or at least allowed to be created for him. The world he inhabits during his physical lifetime is not primarily the physical world as it is, or as it was created, but a world created out of his own mind. What he sees around him with his physical sight, and the sense-impressions he receives, are interpreted by this mental structure which forms the basis for all he takes as real.

Every person born into a physical body is born into an established cultural pattern of one kind or another; he acquires a certain kind of mentality from his family and, later on, from his school and the larger social context in which he finds himself.[10] Apart from this social-cultural mind which each person in a sense inherits at birth, everyone without exception brings with him into a physical life experience *his own mind*. This is his own unique form of Etheric Substance which has been worked upon by his own evolving will, the forms of which were created over many periods of existence on other etheric planes. Every person comes into the physical world with this etheric reality which is unique to himself and will pre-structure all his experience on the physical/material plane. Each person arrives with a mind that also contains accurate memory-traces of his previous existences which, however, usually remain inaccessible to him during his physical lifetime.[11] This is partly because of the way in which his physical mind becomes structured, but it is due even more to the kind of etheric mind he has built up over long periods of time. Most people are at the stage where their minds are built on more or less rigid conceptions of *what is*, this absolutistic rather than relative structuring having been built up in their minds long before entering upon physical life on earth. It is *through* these mental structures that the new physical life is experienced and upon them that all new impressions are received.

If the *a priori* nature of mind is not recognised by most men, it is mainly because by the nature of his mental structure, which he has built up through successive experiences, *man views each current life as the only life he has ever experienced*. This very structure of mind excludes any sense of the continuity of life or the possibility of different life-expressions; it tends to repress or exclude any form of feed-back or inspiration from knowledge acquired in previous 'lifetimes', except indirectly. For most people on earth, knowledge about 'eternal life' or spiritual growth through continuous life-expressions does not form part of their mind-structure when they come into physical bodies. They do not bring with them minds which are structured to accept the existence of more than one life – even though they have in fact already experienced numberless forms of life over a vast period of time. Each form of life has constituted for them the only life, either end of which fades into shadowy existence. In between existences, so to speak, in these shadowy wings, there is a fading out of memory so that each 'on-stage' call appears like an original 'first night'.[12]

And yet, traces of personal etheric memory reach the

consciousness of nearly everyone at some point during the physical lifetime. These memory-traces from previous life-expressions remind people in a fleetingly tantalizing manner of a place once visited, a familiar experience or condition, or of an intimate relationship beneath what currently appears casual or superficial. Few people are completely without an experience of 'déjà vue', and yet few people understand its nature or are able to bring any one of these experiences into focus because the mind in which they live is too limited and its terms of reference too narrow to incorporate an understanding of what these traces of memory mean. The minds which most people inhabit could not accommodate any real knowledge of previous existences, except in a fanciful way which explains them, for example, in terms of *having been* a particular – often historical – person in a previous life.[13]

Each person within Creation is on a certain etheric or mental level which, at any one time, defines reality for him whether his life is being pursued in a physical or an etheric body. The kind of body he is momentarily inhabiting does not in itself alter his mind or what he takes as real. The only possibility of change in his kind of reality – that is, a fundamental change in what he sees and experiences as real – is through a change of mind. Change in the kind of reality a person experiences comes only through an acceptance of the fact that the mind is the seat of his experience of reality, and it comes then only through a strong desire on the part of his will to experience new aspects of reality. This desire must be pursued consciously until experience loosens instead of reinforces the old structure and old forms, and truly *new* experience becomes possible. Each mind can be cleansed in time so that all its forms *reflect* etheric reality truly instead of limiting or distorting it. This is not only a possibility but a goal towards which all spiritual growth is tending. But this can only take place after a man has accepted that the reality he thinks he sees is in fact the mind he inhabits and, recognising this fact, takes responsibility for his mind by questioning every form it contains.

II

Etheric reality and the different levels of which it is made up may be represented diagrammatically as a *ladder* consisting of fourteen rungs. The seven upper rungs represent the stages or levels through which man progresses, through limitless experience and uncountable lifetimes, towards ever-increasing understanding and awareness. The seven lower rungs stand for the corresponding levels of distortion and lead from relatively minor states of mental distortion to a state of all-encompassing spiritual darkness. Although the rungs lead downwards in the sense that they represent states of decreasing light, they do *not* stand for any possible retrogression for man. A man cannot retrogress by descending through levels of darkness in the same way he can *progress* and grow towards increasing consciousness and understanding. A man can descend into only one state of distortion at a time, the level of which depends upon the negative forms he has allowed to develop in his own being. From this state he does not retrogress further into still lower states, but, after much help from others and through his own efforts, he can return to the state – or stage – from which he came. His return to this state never involves a progression upwards through lesser states of distortion. The healing of each 'illness' – and these lower states can best be thought of as forms of spiritual illness – means a return to a state of relative health, not a long progression through other kinds of illness. For each of the seven lower states of distortion is in fact distinct in itself and corresponds only to the particular mental form of which it is an aberration; it does not actually relate to the other lower levels as to rungs on a ladder.

Each of the seven *lower* stages is a distortion, in some respects, of the corresponding *upper* level or stage of growth. Thus, the first level downwards corresponds in a certain way to the first level on the ascending ladder, and the second level downwards represents a distortion of the second level on the ascending ladder, and so on. The highest etheric level – where Mind may be compared to a pure crystal, which *truly* reflects all life and where a man's consciousness includes the whole etheric sphere – has a corresponding level of distortion which is a place of rock-like density, to which the breath of spiritual life and growth can only with difficulty penetrate. But the correspondence of a particular level of distortion with an ascending level is descriptive, not specific or personal, and does not relate to the lives of individual men and women. A person on the second level of evolution, who allows himself to be drawn into a particular state of distortion, does not necessarily descend to the second lower level; nor does someone on the third level find that his own form of distortion leads automatically onto the third lower level. Each *kind* of state finds its correspondence in a particular *place* on the descending ladder, but there is no inherent correspondence between the kinds of distortion and the evolutionary level of a person's being. It is furthermore only possible for people on the *first four* rungs of the evolutionary 'ladder' to descend into states of distortion and places of darkness; after that a man arrives at the level from which such a descent is no longer possible for him.

The life of every man, whether he is in a physical or an etheric body, depends on the level he inhabits. Each level has its own dimensions, and the experiences of those who inhabit a particular etheric level cannot extend beyond its boundaries,[14] and usually are contained within only a small segment of it. The manner in which a person experiences the 'reality' he sees, the structure of his knowledge: in other words, the *totality* of his life, is limited by the etheric plane on which he lives. The upper levels, however, always include the evolutionary levels beneath them, through which the person has already passed.

For most people, the etheric level or plane on which they live represents a limitless area, with vast unexplored and even unimagined regions. The experiences, knowledge, understanding, conception of 'reality' of a single individual on any one level are usually confined within very narrow limits; the boundaries of his particular plane are far distant and there is much to explore and learn before there is any possibility of moving on to another, higher etheric level. In fact, there can be no move at all until the person has exhausted all the opportunities to which his own will could attract him, and learned all there is to learn on any one level. He has to become conscious of his life and his own mind *where he is* before he can begin to move on to another level.

Movement exists on and within every level; everything is in movement, nothing within the earth's etheric is at rest. For man also there is constant movement; there is no *rest* for man, his mind is either expanding or it is contracting. (Rest is not synonymous with passivity, nor is it the same as relaxation; motion or movement is not the same as activity or tension. Motion includes an alternation of activity and passivity.) On every level there is the possibility of either expansion or contraction for man. For man alone exists the possibility of vertical movement. Wherever he is in the etheric sphere, choice exists from moment to moment of affirming either upwards or downwards; from every point in the etheric there is an upwards and a downwards movement – *for man alone.* Choice depends upon a degree of consciousness appropriate to his own level, for choice involves a man's will. When a person makes a choice he begins to take responsibility for his life; it may be the 'wrong' choice, but the fact of choosing at all means he has come to the point in his own evolutionary pattern where he sees his life as capable of being structured by himself.

Choice only exists after a certain stage has being reached. When a man's choices tend 'upwards' he begins to spiritualise his life and everything and everyone related to it. This is the way of spiritual growth and change in level of mind, reality, and being.

From what has been called the 'Summerland' there are six further etheric levels that extend upwards with ever-increasing degrees of consciousness. In certain respects these seven levels resemble the rungs on a ladder, but not every rung – or level – is entirely discrete or separate from all the others. The first four etheric levels constitute, in fact, a single vast sphere, within which movement is gradual and slow-growing; the fifth level is a separate sphere and represents a discrete evolutionary step; the sixth and seventh levels together constitute a single sphere, separate from the preceeding fifth level and within which progression is through manifold stages. Thus, the whole universe of man's etheric evolution consists of three vast spheres with expanding levels of experience, mentality, and consciousness. The first sphere contains the first four levels through which man evolves; the second and smaller sphere consists of the fifth and transitional level; and the third sphere comprises the two highest etheric levels of being. Each person inhabits the portion of that sphere which is appropriate to his own stage or level of mind. Movement for any person is possible only within that portion of the sphere he inhabits, to which the dimensions of his own mind approximate; movement throughout the whole of any sphere exists only for those people who have evolved through all its different stages. All people living within the same sphere are visible to one another in their etheric forms, but their etheric *natures* are not visible except to those who exist on a higher level of consciousness.[15] People on the fourth etheric level, for example, appear as 'beings of light' to those on the first level, but the *nature* of their beings is not apparent to them.

The Summerland may be thought of as a kind of reception centre for everyone who passes out of physical life and whose being corresponds to any one of the first four etheric levels. All awaken into a summer-land of reality which, like its name, gives off a radiance and vibration of sensual experience that exceeds the highest dreams and most vivid imaginings of the physical mind. Every desire, from the flightiest to the most earnestly-harboured longing, finds fulfilment there *according to the nature of the person's being*. The Summerland is, in a sense, a place of infinite response to request. If someone desires food and drink, he is able to obtain the greatest delicacies. And he may continue to eat and drink until he comes *in his own time* to the realisation that such sustenance is no longer necessary for him and another kind of desire supercedes this one. (If food and drink had been an obsession with him during his physical lifetime – if he were gluttonous or dissolute, he would not be in the Summerland but on a lower level of reality.)

Every real desire or longing that has remained hidden in a person during his physical lifetime is revived after his passing and finds expression in the Summerland; here he can learn to paint or play a musical instrument, study any subject in any field of learning, or engage in any activity which is either new or familiar to him. If he were a gardener in his physical life, he may continue to garden and find new scope and new expressions under different and easier conditions. If he had been a librarian, he might pursue his work in the vastly extended libraries and places of learning in the Summerland. Anyone concerned with the discovery of Truth, in whatever form, can find at last those infallible Records of true human history which will quench all thirst for Knowledge. Opportunities exist for every possible form of learning or activity and they are open to everyone. If the desire is present, the person soon discovers the way to its fulfilment. There is response to every *harmless*[16] request in a way undreamed of in physical life, where physical and material limitations structure the form and degree of every response.

There are limitations, however, even in the Summerland. Not all responses to request are in accordance with the person's imagination about himself and his needs – although they are *always* in response to that conception of reality upon which the person's being (or feeling of 'I') is based. All responses operate in accordance with a law of Affinities or Correspondences. This means that the person receives according to the nature of his own being. For example, his 'house' in the Summerland – and everyone in the Summerland finds that a dwelling of some sort awaits him – corresponds to the kind of *mental environment* in which he lived while on the physical plane. It contains the things he loved or gave attention to, and much that gave him pleasure in that life. But it is also furnished with the dark and miserable and distorted, if these were the thoughts he inhabited during his physical lifetime. His etheric home is a reflection of, or embodies, his old familiar self because it is his *home*; it is an externalisation of all that he has valued or cared about, and of the place he occupied in his mind. If it contains dark corners or places filled with mould and bird droppings, it is because these represent the thoughts with which his mind was occupied. His etheric home can never be the embodiment of an abstraction or fantasy but reflects truly the state of his own being.

The central meaning of the Summerland – the key to its existence both as an etheric reality, to be experienced most fully by people who are not in physical bodies, and as a level of mentality which a person may inhabit during physical life on earth as well – is *longing* or *desire to have* and its fulfilment. A person's *desire to have* something for himself, whatever it may be – providing it does no harm etherically either to himself or others, finds fulfilment in the Summerland. It may be for parties and birthday cake, skill in playing the violin, or the opportunity to study the structure of minerals. The meaning central to these and the most varied expressions is the desire *to have*: to have enjoyment, to have proficiency, to have knowledge. If the mind of a person *centres* around any kind of desire to have something for himself, whether material or non-material, then he already inhabits the Summerland, even if he is currently entered upon physical life on earth, and he will, in time to come, receive every opportunity to give fullest expression to his desire.[17] If the desires are of a material nature, he will find a response on this level[18] until such time as he is satisfied and the nature of his desires changes. Summerland is the land where 'missed opportunities' and unfulfilled desires from a person's physical life find expression and satisfaction. It is also the land where each person's desires and enjoyments can undergo gradual transformation and spiritualisation as his own being, through the learning process of these experiences, becomes increasingly refined in its nature.

People inhabiting the Summerland are at widely divergent stages in their own patterns of growth. Some people may be at the commencement of their own evolution and have vast periods of experience to undergo before the desire to move on to a stage beyond that of *desiring to have* or possess takes shape in them. There will also be people in the Summerland whose beings have already evolved to the frontier of the next stage but who still feel they are 'missing' one thing or one opportunity, and who need to remain where they are to give expression to this one desire before the impetus to move on is complete in them.

The next stage in the evolution of a person's being and mind, after all desires *to have* have been expressed and satisfied in the form peculiar to each individual, may be described as the desire for *self expression*. Out of the desire to express, the self develops, in the course of a person's evolution through this second level, the desire to create forms, and, finally, the desire to find self fulfilment in some form of service to other people. Thus, the second level contains many aspects of self expression and people who are at vastly different stages in the evolution of their desires for self expression. Only after a man has gone through numerous forms of self expression does the will to express *for* other people, or to become active in the service of others, begin to take root and grow in him.

The condition of a person who has acquired something – that is, the more passive state of satisfaction which may be reached again and again in the Summerland – soon becomes one of satiety and is a condition in which few people can remain for long, whether during physical life or life on an etheric plane. Minds soon become restless and desire activity through seeking other goals, pursuing other aims. This impetus to change: to activity, movement, and, eventually, to spiritual growth, is inherent in the nature of man, as distinct from all other forms of Creation. In his own time, and sometimes only after long ages of seeking down many different paths, a man arrives at the frontier of a new country of activity, beyond the Summerland. This country is characterised by the *desire to express himself*: to express the experiences he has had and out of which his self has been built up or constituted. Every desire for self expression, every desire to create, belongs to this new stage, this second level of etheric reality.

When the person arrives at this new stage, limitless opportunities again open out before him. His life changes because his aim in life has altered – because the motive force within his own will, in terms of which he sees and hears and pursues his life, is no longer the same. Although he continues to live in the Summerland in one sense, he is no longer *of it* in the same way; his eyes are open to new aspects of it which he did not notice before when he was pursuing his own interests from the desire to have or acquire. He can now see other people and their activities in a different light; in fact, people inhabiting the first etheric level may now become transparent to him mentally. Their thoughts, emotions, motives, and their aims can become increasingly visible to him. However, they do not see any change in him. He will appear to them the same person he always was, except for the fact that he may be engaged now in some other activity in which they do not share; he doesn't seem to have as much time for them as previously: he is moving out of their orbit or place of habitation. In this way he begins to inhabit a new etheric or mental country.

Some occupations in the Summerland can open out more rapidly onto this new level of activity for the people engaged in them, without any real consciousness of change[19] or movement on their part. They will be doing what is already natural to them and something which they learned during their physical life – or even before that, on the etheric plane of a previous existence. The teacher, doctor, social worker – the list of possible occupations and professions is long – is concerned with some form of service to others, although not everyone who engages in any one of these occupations is motivated by the desire to serve or even the desire for self expression. The *desire to have or acquire* may be the primary motivation, whatever the 'profession' or activity in which the person is engaged. But when a person stops looking at the world through the eyes of what it can give him and begins to see it instead from his own *desire for self expression* and, later on, from a sense of what he can give it, then the world itself changes for him. He is no longer where he was: either in himself or in the kind of reality he inhabits.

The Creative Artist, whatever the nature of his work, belongs to the second etheric level. Many people go through this stage of creative activity, whether on a physical or an etheric plane; but it does not belong to everyone's pattern of evolution. There are many degrees of creativity, extending from the beginning stages of the second level to its furthermost boundary with the next etheric level. But everyone who engages in *creative* activity at all has already evolved beyond the *desire to have* for himself and has become sensitive to other desires moving within him – even if they are as yet only vague intimations of a new direction. It is from – or through – these inner promptings or desires, which indicate a new growth of will, that the material as well as the impetus for his creative activity derives. The person himself may look on his creative activity only as forms of *self* expression and fail to recognise the fact that creative activity involves not only an expression of thought, desire, and motive from within (that is, an expression of *intuition*), but also the desire to communicate these intimations of within-ness with other people. This desire to communicate is an integral part of all true creative activity; it is one of the earlier stages in the evolution of the desire to serve others. Without this desire to communicate what is *within* to other people, through the medium of particular forms, there can be no real creative activity.[20] In the course of time, through many different kinds of experience, the desire to serve becomes increasingly refined in the Creative Artist. He may become more and more a vehicle for the expression of those forms and symbols which encourage and help other people in their own spiritual evolutions. But to become such a vehicle, the Creative Artist must evolve in will and consciousness himself to the point where his desire to serve the spiritual needs of others predominates over the desire for mere *self expression*. When he reaches this stage, at the frontier of the second etheric level, his intuitions will have become clear and distinctly formed and there will be a direct flow into the shapes he consciously creates in colour, material, or sound-vibration.

On this second etheric level are to be found all the people who have begun to think and act from the desire and will to serve others in whatever occupation or activity they have chosen to engage in. This takes place in the higher stages of the second level, when the desire for self expression becomes transformed into self expression *for others*, and the direction of a person's activity begins to alter accordingly.

Service on behalf of others, as it evolves on the second etheric level, is directed to people who are in the Summerland and on the second level.[21] In fact, the administration of *all* the needs and activities, which constitute life on these two etheric planes, is carried out by people who are evolving through the second level. This includes ministering to the new arrivals in the Summerland – those who have newly shed their physical bodies and need help in one form or another: rest, treatment, comfort, before they can enter fully upon a new existence.[22] The maintenance of this vast etheric world, consisting of the first two levels of evolution, is the responsibility of those who are evolving through that stage of the second level where they are willing and desirous to serve. From the one who tends the gardens to the doctor in the 'rest home', all who are in service, although responsible in the first place to themselves and having freedom to express their own wills, are nonetheless under the direction of ones from a yet higher level. These persons are in control of and ultimately direct all activities on the first two etheric levels; but each person in service – like everyone on *all* etheric levels – has complete freedom of will to accept or reject this direction and even to carry out an activity in his own way. (He is, however, *always* prevented from causing harm of any kind to another person.)[23]

The dimensions of the Summerland lie in a different *plane of being* to those of the second and succeeding etheric levels. A new growth in being, a new point of departure, is necessary before a man can leave the Summerland and enter upon a different kind of life. *Externally* he may still inhabit the same place, although his mind has become differently structured and his *experience* of the place is different to what it was before. No external gulf exists between the Summerland and the second level, nor is there any barrier between the second and third levels; but as each etheric level is constructed on the basis of different mental dimensions, so each one may be said to express a different plane of being. People move through every plane of being in their own time, expressing in their own unique growth-patterns the meanings which characterise the particular plane. So a man grows in relation to the second level from the initial stages of self expression, through his own forms of creativity, to the development in him of the desire to use these forms of self expression in the service of others. In this way, after many kinds of experience and often long periods of time, the person reaches the further borders of the second etheric level and the frontier of a new plane of being.

The third etheric level is, in certain respects, a place that exists and functions parallel to the second level for it is inhabited by people who are also performing a service, but of another kind. These are people who have experienced and passed through that stage of service to others which characterises the second level; so the third plane may be thought of as both an extension of the second level and a place of growth in consciousness and understanding beyond it. As self interest recedes and the desire for self expression becomes redirected towards serving others, so the ability of the person to learn more about the true nature of people's needs and what is possible for them increases. One of the principal characteristics of someone on the third etheric level is the desire to increase the value of his service to others through an extension of his own knowledge, not only about the particular person or persons he is helping but about the nature of human life in general, its structure, origins, aims – and about the nature of the universe in which this life moves and has being. In fact, man's experience on the third plane of being is characterised by his desire to serve the *real* needs of other people rather than merely to use his own forms of self expression in their service. This is the essential difference between the third and second levels.

An increase in knowledge is possible for everyone at every level, whenever a person's desire is strong enough to find expression, because there are Halls of Learning of every kind throughout the entire etheric country. Wherever there is the desire for knowledge, followed by a clear formulation of request, there is always a response *according to the nature of the person's will and the stage of his being.*

Slowly, as both knowledge and sensitivity to other people and to the nature of life grow, the person becomes aware of another kind of work being carried on from this third level, of which he had previously been unaware. This is the work of service to people on the physical earth. This is the focus of all activity on the third etheric level.

The work of service to the physical earth is manifold in its expressions and total in its compass. It covers every possible aspect of physical activity on earth and requires the greatest patience, steadiness of purpose, and intelligence (which means both adaptability and the willingness to learn the principles and techniques for communicating with and helping people in physical bodies) on the part of those who serve. The third etheric level is the lowest level of service to the physical earth;[24] on all the succeeding and higher levels are to be found numerous people engaged in all kinds and degrees of earth work.

The desire to become involved in service to the earth always evolves out of a man's *personal experience* in connection with the physical plane – usually from something which occurred in his own physical life. He may have an overwhelming desire to help someone (or ones) he has known during his own lifetime in a physical body, whose needs he now recognises and understands. In time, this desire to help will become the focal point in his life and he will then attract the persons who can instruct him in how to commence his work of service to the earth. Sometimes a man is contacted by friends or family already working on this etheric plane, who can help him and with whom he may be able to work. There are many rightful ways and paths along which the person desiring to help someone can be guided when he has reached the appropriate stage in his own evolution.

One kind of personal experience which, in time, can inspire a person with the desire for earth service is the need to rectify or put right some train of events, casual sequence, harm or distortion which he has brought about – intentionally or unintentionally – during his own life in a physical body. For there awakens in everyone, in the course of time, the desire to help in some way the ones he harmed or to state the truth where he had previously conveyed a deception. When this desire becomes the strongest motive in a person's life, the opportunity will be presented for service to the physical earth.

A third way in which the desire to serve the physical earth may awaken in a person is through the profession in which he worked during his own physical life or which he has taken on since his arrival on the etheric plane. For example, a doctor may desire to use his professional skill in the service of people who are still in physical bodies or to collaborate, from the etheric plane, with colleagues working on the physical plane.[25] When this desire becomes the overriding one in a person's life, the opportunity is presented for its fulfilment – but usually only after some period of preparation.

This is the personal basis out of which all work on the earth plane commences on the third etheric level and from which all subsequent work evolves. In part it is concerned with a deepening or spiritualising of the physical experiences and relationships of the people involved. But it is not until a person reaches the third level in his own evolution that this work can be undertaken for the benefit of all concerned.

The journey towards higher states of consciousness and wholeness of being, which man thinks of in terms of *at-onement with God* – the god within – commences on the third etheric level. It starts from the desire and willingness of a person to accept his own life (in all its previous forms) and become responsible for it and all the relationships connected with it. If this stage begins while he is still in a physical body he can journey forward more rapidly than is possible for him on a purely etheric plane of existence, through assuming additional forms of responsibility towards people with whom there is no apparent personal connection. In this way, the person arrives eventually at the fourth etheric level. He never grows to this point through solitary meditation or the performance of spiritual gymnastics of any kind, but solely through taking on increasing degrees of responsibility for himself, the relationships in his life, and towards all other forms of life around him.

This gradual movement from the third to the fourth level of reality comes about through a simultaneous growth in a person's consciousness and in his ability to take responsibility. This may occur while the person is still in a physical body, but it usually takes place more slowly after he has passed on to another form of life on the etheric planes. It commences when the person begins to take on additional responsibilities without neglecting his more *personal* relationships. But gradually the desire to 'personalise' experience lessens and his own involvement or relationship with people becomes less personal, in the sense of being less self oriented, and therefore more *real*. He begins to learn what is possible and desirable for *them* as individuals and so there is less of his own self will in his activities on their behalf. This does not mean that his old relationships die or become 'cold', but a new quality of *concern* enters into them which is not possible so long as they are dominated by his self will. This new *concern* comes from his Heart Centre – it is the first intimation of the awakening Heart Centre from which a new kind of growth becomes possible – and is guided by his Head Centre and its intuitions; it is not connected with the *personal self*[26] which still desires its own expression and satisfaction in every relationship. A move to the fourth level of reality means, in fact, the beginning of a shift in emphasis within the person from the personal to the non-personal. Personal relationships – the personal self and its desires – do not fade away completely at this stage; but the centre of balance for the person on the fourth etheric level becomes in time a new quality of concern for the true nature and potentiality in other people, which in-forms and guides the person's awareness and activities.[27]

Greater responsibilities, on a far larger scale, become possible for the person who is evolving on the fourth etheric level. These responsibilities may be directed towards the higher administration of the first and second etheric levels, for all direction and administration of these first two levels comes from the fourth level – as does all work for the help and regeneration of people on the first four 'lower' levels. (All missions to these four lower spheres are directed from the fourth etheric level.) A person on this fourth level may also have responsibilities on the physical plane of earth, where he can organise and carry out special missions concerned with the healing or protection of large numbers of people. He may also be engaged in the vast missions of 'rescue work' for people who experience either violent or 'unprepared' death and who are unable to accept or comprehend the 'new conditions' in which they find themselves.

All missions from this level are self initiated and stem from both the personal desire and the non-personal concern of individuals at this level, although every help or aid is placed at the disposal of anyone seeking to take responsibility for any kind of mission. There is no 'higher authority' to control them or interfere unless harm is being done in any way to others, in which case the mission would be withdrawn (by persons from a still higher level) and the person responsible would be drawn to the lower level appropriate for acting out his experience and learning the consequences of his actions. Such a removal to a lower level would be in no sense *retributive*, for there is no such thing as retribution on any etheric level that resembles, in any way, the systems of judgment and penal retribution devised by men on the physical plane. (All conceptions of harsh, retributive justice derive, in fact, from the lower levels and are the invention of human distortion.) A person 'falls' through his own choice, and is attracted to a lower level according to the law of affinity: of like attracting like, not because of any punishment meted out to him by a 'higher authority'. It is only through the Law of Protection that missions can be interfered with which endanger the spiritual natures of other people. This is a law[28] which operates on all the etheric[29] levels through which man evolves, including the Summerland, and predicates that no one – indeed, no form of life – is allowed to suffer through the actions of another. A person may *unintentionally* cause harm to another, in which case he immediately becomes aware of it through experiencing in himself what he has caused the other to experience. (This also applies in cases of unintentional suffering caused to animal or plant life.) This law operates on all the etheric levels that lead towards growth of being. If the person perseveres in causing suffering, he becomes involved in doing harm *wilfully* to another. (He might not think of it as 'harm' or imagine that the 'end justifies the means'.) If this happens, he is attracted through his actions to a lower level where this law does not operate and where he can pursue his activity with impunity, until such time as he becomes truly aware of what he is doing and desires change and betterment with his whole being.

From the third or fourth etheric level onward people can be chosen as spiritual companions to accompany those who are about to enter upon physical life on earth, remaining with them throughout the whole of that life. The role of the spiritual companion[30] is to protect, guide, inspire, and instruct the person whom he accompanies so that he can make the best possible use of physical life for his own spiritual evolution. All people born into a physical body from any of the normal etheric levels, including the Summerland,[31] have spiritual companions[32] who accompany them throughout their entire physical lives. Even people who have, from their own free wills, elected to be born ahead of time – before the time intended for their physical experience (that is, the best time from the point of view of their spiritual evolution) – have spiritual companions if they are born with normal (i.e., not distorted) minds.[33] But people who are born from the lower spheres, with some form of mental distortion, do not necessarily have spiritual companions assigned to them from birth.[34]

III

It is in the very nature of the human creation that no one can remain static; but perpetual movement for the human being, unlike the other forms of creation, does not only mean movement in one place but linear movement: growth, evolution – and, frequently, retrogression. The inner being of every man (which is his divine will), working in the etheric medium on either the physical or the etheric plane, is restless and longing, impelling him continuously towards greater consciousness, increased understanding, a larger sense of responsibility. However long the man dallies or delays, the being within him never ceases from its restless probing, searching, and will always break through the limits within which it confines itself from stage to stage.

This is true at all stages in a man's evolution, from the lowest to the highest. When he reaches the outermost limits of the fourth level of reality, so the same restless desire of his will makes itself felt eventually by breaking through every position of responsibility which the person has built up and forcing upon him a new beginning.

By the time a person has reached the latter states in his evolution through the fourth level, two centres of gravity have become fully developed in him. One is the old *feeling of 'I'*, centred around his desire for self expression, which has evolved through many phases, expressed through many forms, and become formulated as a 'self' over vast periods of time that involved many kinds of experience. The second centre of gravity begins to form in a person when he is still on the third level of reality, around a growing sense of responsibility towards people with whom he has no *personal* relationship. It develops more fully on the fourth etheric level as a new focal point in the experience or feeling of *concern* connected with the person's Heart Centre and postulates a *non-personal* yet caring relationship to other people and to the whole living world around him. By the time the person has reached the furthermost frontier of the fourth level, these two centres of gravity co-exist in him, equal to one another in significance and strength and therefore creating, for the first and only time, a real dichotomy of interest, desire, and will. For there are many times when the two poles in him are in basic disagreement over aim and direction. There is no other point in the whole etheric evolution of man when such inner dualism exists. This is a stage to which every person comes at the appropriate time in his own evolution and through which experience of tension, and often confusion, he has to go. For neither centre of gravity is capable in itself of outweighing the other; the desire or will that is reflected in *concern* or *caring* can never become strong enough in itself to overshadow the self, with its long history of experience, and dominate its desire for expression. After a long period of time – the exact measure being appropriate to each individual's pattern of growth, when the tension has become almost unbearable, a third factor enters into the experience of the person, silently and at first almost imperceptibly. This is the point at which the person enters upon the fifth level of reality.

This new factor which has awakened within the man, making possible his entrance upon a new and discrete level of experience, is the *desire for at-onement with God*. This is the central focus of meaning for all life and all experience on the fifth etheric level; for every individual the fifth level becomes a spiritual journey towards at-onement.

Every experience and all forms and expressions of life that existed on the fourth level continue to exist on the fifth level as the media through which each individual journeys at this stage. He does not leave or neglect the forms of activity which structured his life in the latter stages of the fourth etheric level, but they become centred around a new motivation which is his search for God. He does not reject the forms of mind which delineated all his thinking, but they become for the first time not so much *tools* as objects to be searched for clues or waymarks on the journey. Everything in the person's life becomes part of his search, upon which the intensity of his longing for God becomes focussed. The urgency of this desire for God in a person eventually supercedes completely, if only temporarily, both the desire for self expression and the sense of *caring* or *concern* which had formerly existed in him as a dichotomy of opposing wills.

At no other stage in the evolution of man is there a spiritual journey of this nature, for at no other stage – on no other level before this one – is man *one-centred* in his desire or will, purpose, and direction. Religious writings – particularly Christian and Gnostic – and the literature of the mystics contain many descriptions of journeys, but none is the journey of man at this stage in his evolution. Some of them use a sexual imagery which relates to another aspect of life altogether. Many form part of a particular religious tradition, expressing its terminology and structure of belief. But the true spiritual journey, when it takes place at the right moment in every man's pattern of evolution, is contained within no religious form of any kind and expresses no doctrinal beliefs or particular faith; for all religious forms belong at their highest to the fourth etheric level and many belong to an experience of the Summerland or to the lower levels. The spiritual journey is not formal or ritualistic; there is no established pattern for its expression, no archetypal structure for it to follow. *Each* spiritual journey is unique and expresses within the individual's experience and relationships; and the person derives from this journey a 'treasure' which is uniquely his own.

The life of the person becomes immensely simplified in the course of his journey through the fifth level – and refined or purified of all that is superfluous to his search for God. For, in time, this search lights up each experience and every relationship which belongs to the whole of the person's etheric life, and in the process of clarification the irrelevant and the less important gradually disappear.

The fifth level of reality may be thought of as a place of transition, an intermediate country between two very different spheres or two fundamentally different kinds of mentality. It is a bridge between the world of *subjective* realities and the world of *objective* reality, where the desire or will to find God, in order to achieve what may be called *mystical union* (or Samadhi), becomes transformed slowly into the search for Truth. When the desire for Truth becomes so formed in the individual that it is the focal point in every experience and in all relationships, then he has entered upon the sixth etheric level.

The search for God – the desire for mystical union – which grew out of the opposition between two different expressions of will in a person, becomes transformed into the search for Truth within the *practical* context of his life, within its pattern of activity. It can never come about through an artificial withdrawal from life into some form of contemplative state.[35] When this desire to find God is expressed in the midst of experience (whatever the nature of that experience) or in a relationship, God becomes the touchstone of Truth within that experience or relationship. God, being within the experience, reveals to the person its true nature and meaning. In this way God gradually becomes Truth for the person; imperceptibly, over a long period of time, his search for a personal God becomes transformed into a search for non-personal Truth.

The experience of Truth transcends and brings together in the person the two different and often opposing expressions of his will. The Truth reveals to him both the nature of his *caring* or *concern* and the structure of the self and its desire for expression which had evolved over vast periods of time. The search for God, which marked his entrance into the fifth etheric level, becomes the search for and receptivity to Truth at its further border with the suceeding level of reality; and the desire for mystical union, or *Samadhi*, is transformed through living experience into a re-uniting or making whole of his entire being. For as Truth reveals to him *what is*: its history and structure, its purpose and direction, so every facet or aspect of his being falls into perspective and finds that place in which it can serve most usefully his expression of life in the highest etheric sphere.

The sixth and seventh levels of reality comprise a single sphere in which the experience of Truth gradually reveals to man the nature of his own being and the true nature of the whole etheric universe through which he has evolved, which is its Objective Reality. Truth works in each person who has reached this stage through the mind which has evolved in him, through his own unique experiences. Even at the highest level, there is no *abstract* Truth; for Truth is unique – although not merely *subjective* – with every individual, and each person knows only that part of Objective Reality to which his own experiences give him access and which his mind is therefore able to reflect.

The mind of man is essentially crystalline in structure; it was created with the capacity for becoming many-facetted through experience and, eventually, reflecting Truth as the facets of a crystal mirror the world about it. So long as a man lives through various modes of self expression, experiencing himself as separate and closed off from the world about him, the mind he inhabits is personal to his own desires and will and the world it reflects is also coloured by what is personal to him. His mind cannot truly reflect what is around him, but rather colours and structures all his impressions. It reflects likewise his imaginings and fantasies. When the personal, isolated, and imaginary are transcended, after a long process of evolution, so his mind can begin for the first time to exhibit the nature of its underlying structure, as a special kind of crystal.

All the levels, stages, and aspects of life in the etheric universe, through which a man has evolved, can become reflected in the crystal of his mind, as if in a mirror, once the distorting agent of personal identifications and imagination is dissolved. But this is not achieved in the 'twinkling of an eye'; it is the ultimate goal of a process which commences on the sixth etheric level and extends throughout the entire sphere to the highest stage at the seventh level. The achievement of a mind structured like pure crystal is the work of long periods of time and the goal at the far end of that country through which every man will progress eventually. Such is the ultimate nature of the etheric mind, and this is its purpose: to reflect accurately, truly, and without any personal distortion all that exists in the etheric sphere *which the person has himself experienced*. All thirteen[36] levels of reality are then reflected in this mind.

In order to understand the significance of this *reflective mind* it must be seen in relation to the preceding stages in the growth of mind. At the first stage, individual mind forms part of group mind and possesses little independence of expression and choice. This stage exists on the etheric plane as well as among so-called primitive people on the physical plane. The second stage in the evolution of mind is delineated in terms of personal like and dislike or desire and rejection. A man's awareness of the world around him at this stage is largely defined by these categories and his awareness of himself is comprised largely in terms of states ranging from happy to depressed, according to the world's response to his personal desires. Endless impressions of all kinds from the world about him impinge on his being, but his mind receives them on this structure of personal 'desire and rejection' and his awareness extends very little beyond it.[37]

This stage of mind, or kind of mentality, extends throughout the first two etheric levels which every man has to live through and experience, in various ways, for a long period of time. Even on the second level, where a man is no longer totally absorbed in seeking pleasure or interests for himself – or in self expression for its own sake, but has arrived at the stage of concern for other people, this structure of mind still exists but in an *enlarged form*. The scope of his personal 'liking' has expanded with the desire to express himself *for* other people, to use his talents and interests on their behalf. His consciousness now includes the people whom he can 'help' through his own personal forms of self expression; but the *kind* of mentality through which he lives his life on this level remains the same, for it is still determined by personal desires and his actions are moved largely by the same kind of fluctuation in his own states as before.

The third stage in the evolution of man's mind commences with the third etheric level, for this stage is denoted by the re-structuring of mind in terms of *responsibility*. The idea of being responsible for his life and for the people in his life first occurs to the person as a *seed thought* when his mind has expanded to the point of being able to receive it. This seed takes root slowly and grows through many experiences on different planes. When the person's will has wholly responded to this idea of *personal responsibility* then it transcends and ultimately replaces the former structure of mind based on like and dislike, varying desires, and fluctuating emotional states. It is this new mind, formed around the will-to-personal responsibility, that grows eventually into an instrument which the person can use in ministering to others and which now provides a continuity of purpose and effort.

It is through many expressions of service on the third and fourth etheric levels and through the slow growth and expansion of this new mind, on this mental level, that the person begins to form and fashion the various *facets* of his mind. Each kind of experience creates a new *facet* of mind, in much the same way that a sculptor chisels into rock. And each mental *facet*, cut and formed out of the crystal-like potential of mind, represents the 'treasure' harvested from the particular experience, out of the man's perseverance and learning through that experience. Earlier experiences and relationships, which belong to the person's previous evolutionary stages in the Summerland and on the second etheric level – even on lower levels – and are purposefully reworked on the third or fourth levels, form definite *facets* on the person's mind. Each *facet* constitutes an indestructable part of the person's etheric mind, capable, eventually, of reflecting all other similar experiences being undergone by *anyone*, anywhere in the etheric sphere.

Every experience which a man can have, on whatever plane of life, is capable of adding a new *facet* to his mind with which he can then 'see' and understand. But the creation of any *facet* of mind depends, first of all, on his assuming responsibility for the experience, understanding its nature, and working it through completely until the essence of the experience has achieved a certain crystalisation in him. Sometimes the treasures which his mind gathers through many experiences appear in the form of 'gifts' or talents and sometimes they are not visible at all.

The kinds of personal experience, out of which the *facets* of a man's mind are shaped, belong to all the etheric levels up to and including the fifth level. On the two highest levels, experience is no longer personal and does not lead to the formation of new *facets*. But until the mind is fully formed and so long as personal experience is necessary, the person will continue to gather it until the structure of his mind is complete. Then, only, when he has reached the stage where the desire for Truth has absorbed every other desire or will, does another process begin which has as its aim the creation of the fourth level of mentality, or the *reflective mind*. Before this new process can commence, which concerns the cleansing of every *facet* on a person's mind, this mind will have reached its greatest extent as a *personal* mind, having gone through all the experiences which are possible for that individual.

From the sixth level onwards the individual mind becomes perfected. Its structure, having been formed like rock-crystals in the crucible of personal experiences, is fixed and the man's task consists in cleansing and polishing each *facet* so that it accurately reflects *what is*. Then he becomes able to use his whole mind as a perfect tool in the service of all life for which he is responsible.

The two etheric levels, six and seven, form part of a single sphere in which this process of cleansing and purification takes place, through which a man's mind gradually becomes able to reflect, truly, the nature of the etheric sphere and to perform with understanding all the tasks and services which have ever belonged to him, throughout the whole of its extent. The clearer the crystalline nature of man's mind becomes, the greater his consciousness of all things and the more enlarged is his sense of responsibility. Any conception of 'blissful inactivity' as belonging to a higher level of consciousness is totally irrelevant and imaginary.

IV

Much of the work and service of people on the fifth, sixth, and seventh levels is concerned with those who inhabit the seven *lower* etheric levels. This is long and often arduous work, for it can take a considerable period of time before people caught up in distorted forms of mentality are able to begin the process of working their way back to the place from which their natural course of evolution began to deviate. This 'process of working their way back' is different for each person, on each of the lower levels, but all such processes have to do with some form of *coming to life again*. For all the lower levels may be thought of as various forms of spiritual deadness, a kind of animated but lifeless existence – often represented, and sometimes actually seen on the physical plane by people with spiritual sight, as differing degrees of 'darkness'. At each level of distortion, and within each particular manifestation of darkness, the person has to work his own way back gradually to that *spiritual life* which had temporarily been suspended in him.[38]

All the levels 'downwards', towards increasing darkness and more complex or wilful forms of distortion, are *discrete* etheric or mental levels. They do not interpenetrate one another, nor do they represent retrogressive stages through which a person may descend. Each one is related loosely, and only in a certain sense, to the corresponding rung on the ladder of human evolution. Such correspondence is only approximate and does not mean that someone at the fourth level of evolution, for example, would fall automatically to the fourth level of 'darkness', if he allowed his mind to become structured by distortion; he could be drawn down to any level depending on the nature of the distortion. But the correspondence between upper and lower levels, however slight, makes possible a clearer understanding of the nature of those spheres in which people live different kinds of distorted lives.

All persons inhabiting the seven lower levels may be thought of as being *stuck* to something that needs to be broken down before they can again enter the path of spiritual evolution. There are many degrees of attachment or identification; at the lowest levels people's minds may be 'crystallised' into a kind of rock-like rigidity that requires long work and perseverance to break down. There are also differences between the kinds of mentality which hold people bound to states from which no spiritual growth is possible. In all cases, on all the lower levels, the point of rigidity or crystallisation colours and distorts the person's conception of reality to the point where the *place* he inhabits etherically corresponds exactly to the nature of his mind. From the third level downwards the person's mind actually *creates* its own forms of reality which become *objective reality*[39] to the person concerned and those around him who are capable of being influenced by his mind. On every level of distortion people's minds are warped or disfigured in some way; on the lowest levels a mind may be twisted into hideous or grotesque shapes. Since the mind is both *observer* and also what is *observed* – state, as well as place of habitation, the person is able to see only the disfigurement or hideousness of his own mind around him. The life of a person's Inner Being will not be able to find expression in either the fifth, sixth, or seventh spheres of 'darkness'. At the lowest level of all a person is said to be in complete darkness because he is totally cut off, through his own mind, even from the voice of his own conscience.[40]

These are the principal characteristics of life on the lower etheric levels.

The first level of distortion is inhabited by people who are identified with a particular negative, personal emotion. This emotion has become a kind of block in the person and cannot easily be altered by any change in the circumstances or conditions of his life. Not even the death of his own physical body will necessarily alter this negative formation in his mind. In many cases, but not all, the negative emotion is caused initially by an experience which occurs during physical life and the person's mind creates forms which assure its perpetuation as a stumbling block beyond the death of the physical body. Identification with a particular emotion and its complex of mental forms means that the person inhabits etherically the *place* to which his kind of mentality corresponds.

The constellation of mental forms is created slowly, over a period of time, while a particular emotion becomes a kind of *focus* in the person's life. The emotion is sometimes the result of a nodal experience in his life – that is, the way he relates to that experience – and it acts as a magnetic pole, attracting to itself related experiences until there is a complex structure of interconnected forms that evoke and reinforce the primary emotion. All the person's experiences are eventually coloured by this unresolved structure of emotion and mental forms.[41] Help from another source – from other people – is usually needed before the bonds of emotional identification are broken and the person becomes free and able to return to his normal form of existence.

Many forms of identification on this first level of distortion are centred on the experience of *fear* and the accompanying mental images which have been created partly by the person's own imagination and which evoke and reinforce the original emotion. *Resentment* is another characteristic emotion which can arise in situations involving family relationships; more frequently it is brought with a person when he enters physical life and manifests as a 'predisposition' to feeling wronged or slighted or neglected.

Resentment, like every form of negative emotion, grows and becomes more complex unless it is dealt with in the beginning with reason and understanding and if the person's will does not allow his mind to create different forms of expression. Although the minds of people on this level are not wholly distorted, nor are all their relationships coloured by their negative feeling of 'I', nevertheless, real growth is suspended for them so long as it exists.

The second level of distortion has many similarities with the first; but the point of identification which holds people to this second level of mentality (and reality) is far more comprehensive and rigid than it was for people on the first level. It affects all the person's relationships, colours his entire mind, and ultimately draws on all his energy. If the person is living on the physical plane, it makes him 'absent' to much of life about him and periodically withdrawn into some shadowy existence of his own.[42] The first and second levels of distortion are the only two lower levels which are not completely separate from one another but represent different degrees of intensity of the same mental problem. And the possibility of descent from the first to the second level exists for anyone who shuts out the voice of his own Inner Being or fails to respond to the help which is offered him.[43]

On the second level the whole etheric being of the person can become directed to the expression of one negative emotional complex, this being frequently connected with a feeling of resentment and a sense of having been 'wronged'.[44] In such a case it is not a question of having been wronged in only one aspect of life or in one set of relationships; the person may believe that his whole life has been ruined. The direction of the resentment or grievance is often impersonal: fate or circumstance has ruined his life by placing him in a certain situation, preventing the development of certain opportunities, hindering the acquisition of particular possessions or the expression of other relationships, by depriving him of good health, and so on. It can also take a more *personal* form of expression. Resentment against a parent can draw to itself every other possible grievance until the whole life becomes focussed on this one negative expression and it is the excuse for every failure to act or to *be*.

Discontent is like a virus infection that can spread rapidly throughout the entire body once it has taken hold and absorb all a person's strength and energy. Some people come into their physical lives with an already-formed state of discontent; everything they experience during physical life can reinforce this discontent, unless they become aware that it is their state of mind and not circumstance which is its cause. Only such awareness on the part of the person himself can enable him to use his own will to allow this complex structure to be broken down by the ones who seek to help him and to create new positive forms in its place.

If the person is 'born before his time' – born before the resolution of difficulties which become far more intractable on the physical plane than on the etheric – he 'wastes' the opportunities for evolution which physical life is intended to offer.[15] Most people whose minds are so structured, and who inhabit this lower level of etheric reality, are *not* able to develop an awareness of the true nature of their state of being while they are in physical bodies, and physical life experiences tend to confirm or strengthen the existing structure of mind. An autocratic parent can call it forth; difficult or depressed, narrow or poverty-stricken circumstances in the life can nourish it; and, if the will of the person allows, it can grow into a deep and lifelong bitterness. Partial discontent can become all-embracing through the experience of disappointment or failure – but only if the will of the person allows it to happen. His will almost always *does* allow it, because the will of a person whose mind opens out onto this second level of distortion is subject to the same confusion and distortion of thought and emotion as is his mind.

It is necessary to understand the role of the will at every etheric level, but it is especially important to see what happens to a man's will on this particular level. For on this level the will of the person *allows* his being to become increasingly absorbed by its negative state; it *allows* the confusion of mind to persist and grow, so that in the end he can do nothing except express his discontent or resentment. On all succeeding and more dense levels, the person's will does not merely acquiesce in the negative structure of mind but becomes *actively* engaged in its *creation*. On the second level, however, the person's will usually becomes immobilised so that he is unable to do anything; he can neither seek what is positive nor does he actively *create* negative forms through which to express or experience. This level may in fact be characterised by an *entropy* of the will. This person needs help from outside himself to become free from his mental imprisonment; but it usually takes a long time before such self-inflicted immobility will give entrance to those forms of help which seek to arouse the will and call on it to 'see' and to make effort for itself.[46]

The third lower level is a different kind of place to the first and second levels. It is not a place where people's wills have become helplessly ensnared in an emotional complex from which they cannot extricate themselves, where they may go on for a long time (in and out of a physical body) reliving their fear, resentment, discontent, until their will to make effort is re-awakened, little by little. On the contrary, on the third lower level the person's will is *actively* engaged in creating situations which encourage the expression of the negative forms which structure his mind and with which he is usually obsessed. The person's will actively encourages his identification with resentment, discontent, pride, or jealousy and activates them through every opportunity. The will is active on this level, not passive.

The person whose mind creates the third lower level as an habitation for himself does not *experience* it as any imprisonment or restriction on his life and self expression because he is actively engaged in its creation. It constitutes reality for him and it is true not only for himself but has a certain *objective validity* because it is a creation of *will*, through the agency of his Creative Imagination. This is the primary difference between existence on this level, and the mentalities of which this level is composed, and existence on the two preceeding lower levels. For on the first two levels mental reality is subjective and possesses validity only for the individuals concerned; they are at the mercy of it – although not continuously – but do not actively seek to project it beyond themselves.

The mental structure of a person existing on the third lower level has *objective* reality for him and he sees other people in terms of this 'reality'; he does not seek to *impose* it on others for there is no violence at this stage. No one wilfully does violence to themselves or to other people on this level. But these 'other people', whatever their own levels of being, will find it difficult to disentangle themselves from the web of 'reality' woven about them and to distinguish truth from what is, in fact, fantasy, because it is so compelling.

People who inhabit this kind of mind or lower etheric level manifest an obsessiveness towards other people which is often overpowering and can sometimes injure[47] the minds of those with less forceful personalities or who are more sensitive – and often more highly evolved spiritually. These people also exhibit a strong sense of their own 'rightness', for their reasoning is oriented towards supporting their obsessions whenever necessary – and whatever they may be, and is convincing *on its own terms*. Their thought-processes are always self referential and circular; they begin and end with the particular attitude or obsession with which they are most strongly identified as characterising 'themselves'.

But people inhabiting this kind of mind are not entirely enveloped by their own forms of self absorption; however obsessive their attitudes and expressions, however distorted the conception of reality associated with their obsession, opportunities still exist for a less self oriented kind of expresssion and for another kind of relationship to be experienced. It is possible for other ideas and other conceptions of reality to penetrate the structure of the person's mind.

All people who are experiencing physical life on earth, the nature of whose mentalities opens out onto this particular level, were born with this kind of mind. It is *never* the result of a physical life but always precedes it. Most people born onto the earth with this particular structure of mind are born at the *right time* for themselves, and it can be altered more easily and the person return to a new growing point during his physical lifetime.[48]

So long as a person is still in a physical body and in reasonable health, he or she will manifest other characteristics besides the ones which reflect his particular obsession. Because of these other forms of expression and the nature of physical life on earth, it is easier for him to become conscious of the underlying negative structure of his mind and its obsession while still in a physical body; for he is surrounded by these other points of contact, opportunities, and challenges – often in the form of other people whose minds are very different from his own. If he passes out of physical life before he has become conscious of the nature of his obsession with himself, it becomes more difficult for him because he is then surrounded by an etheric 'reality' which is solely the reflection of his own mental state.

In a certain sense the lower levels should not be thought of as 'levels' at all but rather as places which are distortions of the stages through which man grows. In the Summerland it is possible for people to become 'trapped' in their own desires, their own wanting, or their own frustrations, and this can lead them into a state which is wholly structured by the desire or the frustration.[49] This 'state', which is subjective, corresponds to a certain kind of *place* which was actually *created* by people at lower, more dense levels of existence and constitutes part of the first lower level.[50] The same principle holds true for the other levels.

The transformations which occur in the *will* of the person between the Summerland and the second level of reality and, again, towards the end of the second level are *nodal points* in the growth pattern of all individuals, where the life is not only capable of growth but also of becoming stuck or distorted. At either point a person can enter into a more or less permanent state of mind which corresponds to the place denoted as the 'second lower level', the level of the distorted and paralysed will. The third level of reality, where the evolving person begins his life of service to others, has a more tenuous connection with the 'third lower level', which may be inhabited by people whose obsessions have to do with imagining they have a special mission of service. The state of religious mania also belongs to this level.

These parallels are useful primarily as additional aids to understanding the nature of the *states* or *places* of distortion into which people can allow themselves to fall. But it is important to remember that there is rarely any real link between the *natural* level of a person's being and the state or level to which his distortion can lead him. A person whose *natural* level – that is, the level to which he belongs through individual effort and growth of being – is the second level can fall to *any* state and inhabit any place of distortion or darkness. The same holds true for anyone on any of the first *four* levels. Even on the fourth level, where people attain to a very high degree of personal responsibility for life in the etheric sphere, a person may fall to any one of the seven lower levels. It is only when he has evolved *beyond* the fourth level that distortion of being is no longer possible for him.

The fourth level of distortion is characterised by an all-embracing ego-centricity which excludes the experience of anything that does not refer to the imagined 'self' of that person. He is completely enclosed by this 'self' and the purpose of all relationships becomes the support or enhancement of this self; external etheric 'reality' proceeds from and is a reflection of the self and its requirements. A person who is in this state, and inhabits this place, is obsessed with a single image of himself – a certain imaginary conception of himself – which his will has affirmed and encouraged, although not created. The descent into this all-encompassing imaginary self, through which and in terms of which all experience proceeds, is the primary characteristic of the fourth level of distortion. Self-inflicted violence also begins at this level, for the mental structures, which the person takes as real, do violence to the real nature of his etheric and physical bodies. A person may touch this level or place momentarily through his own states and, in this way, have a shock experience and insight which redeem him before he comes to inhabit the place more and more, or eventually, altogether.

Down to and including the third lower level, distortion exists in the mind of the person and the only damage to the body is of a less serious or temporary kind which is immediately reparable when the mind has been freed and returned to its natural state. On the fourth level, however, damage to both the etheric and physical bodies is of a more serious and permanent nature, and is not easily repaired even after the mind is released from its total self absorption and works its way back to its natural state. The nature of the person's body (physical or etheric or both) has been violated for him to inhabit this level at all, often through sexual perversion[51] or homosexuality,[52] sometimes through a kind of physical as well as mental infantilism, or by athletic exploitation.[53]

These are the more modern forms through which physical and etheric distortions tend to occur. Far more devastating results have come about in the past through the various 'schools' of fakirs, eremites, 'yogis', mystics, fanatics who taught their adherents to do violence to their minds and physical bodies in order to achieve certain spiritual or mental ends, or to acquire psychic powers. They tortured their bodies with nails or fasting and their minds with mental postures until they became disfigured or distorted. All organised religions have taught, in part and at times, that their god(s) requires some form of self-immolation on the part of the follower; to achieve the more sophisticated aim of a 'higher state of consciousness' a more subtle form of self-mutilation, of an emotional or mental nature, is required. *All* teachings which exact from their followers a denial of one or more aspects of their whole being through certain exercises or psychological practices cause *physiological* as well as mental damage of a lasting[54] nature. Such damage affects and causes distortion to the etheric body of the person, but this only becomes apparent when he has passed out of his physical life on earth. The road to 'immortality' which these sects teach is a road to an immortality of distortion and perversion which will require long and arduous work on other planes of existence – including many forms of help from other people – before it is broken down and dispersed and the person becomes capable of a return to his natural state. This is the road to a state of crystallised distortion, an 'immortal thing-ness', and every path that begins with 'self' denial, 'self' sacrifice, or 'self' violation of any kind leads in this direction.[55]

The mental or etheric 'reality' on the fifth lower level is very different in one essential respect from the preceding levels, for it is characterised by violence towards others. This violence may be of a physical or sexual nature; it may be expressed, as it is in pornography, in written or pictorial forms that violate the minds and imagination; or it may be expressed in forms that glorify acts of physical violence. People exist on the fifth, sixth, and seventh levels of distortion *because they have desired power above all else*. They have used their own wills to create mental forms and structures for the manipulation of others and to feed themselves with a sense of power. They have created their own mental and etheric realities. The world in which they live is *their own creation*: an *objective reality* which they seek to impose on others who have the kind of weakness of will which permits it. Through this 'reality' they manipulate and control other people. In fact, and in the end, they are at the mercy of their own creation, for it controls them. The fifth, sixth, and seventh levels of the lower sphere are structured, furnished, and 'peopled' by the creations of those who dwell on them. Demons, evil spirits, and devils are created and willed into existence by the people on these levels for whom they are as 'real' as any naturally created etheric form. (Demons only exist for those who have created them or who, through weakness, acquiesce in their existence.) Before a person can move from this level he has to use this same power of creation to dematerialise every form of demon or evil spirit to which he has given life.

The differences which exist between the etheric or mental 'reality' on the fifth lower level and the kinds of distortion that obtain on the preceding four levels cannot be exaggerated. When the will becomes active on the third and fourth lower levels, it is in relation to a particular point of identification which it seeks to support and justify; or it is in relation to a certain imaginary conception of the self. It is primarily involved in *self* justifying. The imagination of the person is *self* absorbed. From the fifth level of distortion on, however, the desire for power becomes the motive force and the Creative Imagination of the mind is now used by the will to create forms and vehicles for exercising power over others. At this point the violence which is inherent in the distorted will of a person[56] becomes directed not only towards himself but outwards towards others as well. From this level downwards the person does violence not only to himself but to the physical and etheric beings of other people.

Anyone who engages in *any* form of witchcraft may be drawn to this fifth lower level. Certain Tibetan forms of Tantric Buddhism, connected with an older religion and with demonology, belong to this level. Some 'fringe' religions, teachings, and philosophical schools of an 'esoteric', occult, or 'yogic' nature attract people from the fifth or even lower levels to become teachers and leaders. Extremist social or political groupings, outside the main structures of society, also attract some people from the lower etheric levels who are obsessed with a desire to experience power through violence to others, in the name of whatever 'cause' happens to be current at the time. All human societies in the latter half of the twentieth century have become increasingly dominated by people who are on the fifth and even lower etheric levels.

The sixth level of distortion is inhabited by people who systematically torture others, physically or mentally, for whatever reason. These are people in whom the all-encompassing desire for power has become a lust to use that power to inflict pain, to distort minds, and to crush the spiritual beings of other people into submission. This is not merely the will to *destroy life* (which also exists on the fifth level and is expressed in various ways).[57] The will to torture others to the point of abject submission or complete humiliation is of a different nature altogether and one which represents a much lower state of being, enveloped in much greater spiritual darkness. It is, in essence, the will to destroy the spiritual life, the Divine spark, in another person: to force that life – its light – to submit to darkness. All over the world, especially where one group of people is trying to maintain itself in power by the rule of force, this level of darkness manifests itself through human activity.

Another aspect of the lust for power which characterises this level is expressed through people who do violence to young children. This is not merely a form of sexual perversion, as it is thought to be, but a will to violate or crush into submission what is young and full of spiritual life and light.

On the fifth and even sixth levels people do not live *wholly* in their distortions; some parts of their minds are furnished with other images and forms and they can experience kinds of etheric reality which are not distorted by these forms of power-seeking or cruelty. For example, a person's home-life can exist detached from the place of torture which he may inhabit for many of his waking hours; he can walk out of his degraded mentality into another kind of mentality altogether, as he would into another room, where he is capable of expressing kindness and affection to his wife and children and acting in accordance with normal moral standards. This is the hallmark of *schizophrenie*, and it is on the sixth level of distortion that the true schizophrenic mentality exists.

Schizophrenie is a formation of mind which people have created with their own wills before they entered upon a physical existence, while they were still on other, etheric planes.[58] It is constructed systematically, over a period of time, by someone with a very strong will who uses all the power at its disposal to expel from the sphere of activity in which his will is expressing its lust for power every trace of conscience and every idea of Good or concern for others which could in any way limit its fullest expression or operation. With his own will the person constructs[59] a water-tight compartment in his mind, within which every possible amoral expression of his power-lust can be indulged with impunity. When this 'construction' is completed, nothing can intrude upon, restrain, or influence what the will expresses and creates within that compartment. Yet outside this sphere, in the remaining portion of the same person's mind, conscience and a higher reason may still be operative forces.

People who can in fact be called schizophrenic bring this structure of mind already formed into their physical lives. The appearance they present is exactly as described. They may be considerate, moral, honest in their relationships with friends or family – or even with strangers, while at the same time, in all activities related to their 'sealed compartment', there is no act of violence or cruelty or lust in which they may not indulge. These are two completely separate and very different beings[60] within the same man; and each part of the schizophrenic being is valid for the person in its own place.[61]

The seventh and lowest level of 'darkness' is one in which the entire being of the person has become encompassed by the sealed compartment of the schizophrenic; no part of his mind is open any longer to the influence of his own conscience. His will has completely sealed his mind against receiving any guidance or inspiration from within; although his Inner Being continues to function, he cannot receive its messages. All the impressions he receives from without, whatever their nature, that refer to the world about him or to the people with whom he has a relationship fall on a mind that is totally devoid of direction from within and lacks the least contact with its spiritual meaning.

A person on this level of being might give the appearance of any – or every – form of normality, of having normal relationships, of reflecting ethical values in his behaviour, or even of being religious in outlook. The person is capable of *reflecting* any idea or value from outside while he is at the same time incapable of receiving any inner direction from within his own being, or from his spiritual companion or Guardian Angel; so that the ethic from without can receive no response from within and remains a mask, external to the nature of the person and unable to exert an influence on his will.

This level of mind and etheric being is in no sense a development out of the sixth level; it is not merely a step downwards from the schizophrenic mentality into greater 'darkness'. Within the entire sphere of distortion and darkness there is never movement of any kind from level to level, in either direction. In fact, to think in terms of 'sphere' at all is to create a certain misunderstanding, because levels of distortion are better conceived of as referring *primarily* to mind or mentality rather than to *place*.[62] For most people 'place' – that is, where a person's body is in an *external* sense – is very different from 'mind' which is how he thinks and occasionally where he is *internally*. In reality, a person's mind *is* his internal place and, as such, must necessarily affect his *external* place. In time to come it will be understood more widely that the place in which a person lives 'externally' is *in fact* the same place that he inhabits 'internally'.

This mental sphere of distortion and darkness is therefore not a single *place* in the ordinary sense of the word, nor a ladder of different places. It consists of seven separate and unconnected[63] kinds of mental place which constitute reality in both an inner and an outer sense for the people who inhabit them. The idea of levels within this whole sphere of distorted mind conveys the fact of varying distance from the person's *natural* level and of lesser or greater degrees of spiritual darkness, but it is not intended to convey an impression of movement from one to another as if they were rungs on a ladder. In fact, all the separate levels of distortion open out from the Summerland or from any of the first four upper levels. From any one of these four levels, the person can either will his own growth, and so continue his evolution upwards in his own time, or will those forms of destructiveness which lead him in the opposite direction – into entropy or some kind of lifeless or distorted existence on one of the seven levels of 'darkness'. When the person has recognised his situation, wherever he may find himself in this world of shadow, and desires to change his place of mind, working his way back to his own natural level through the aid of his own will and the help of the ones assigned to him, he can still descend into another – and yet another – level of distortion and darkness. At any point on the way of ascent, through the first four levels of evolution, a person may descend again and again through weakness or the inclination of his own will into different places of distortion. He can never descend into precisely the same place twice, but he can be drawn back into inhabiting a different form of the same *level* of 'darkness' in which he had previously existed. This can recur many times until he has worked out every aspect of a particular weakness and is wholly able to will the growth and evolution of his own life. Most people can only learn in this way, through many experiences of descent into places created by weak will, self absorption, or violence of one form or another. A few people are able to learn, overcome their own weaknesses, and grow without such experiences.

Someone who has experienced 'crystallisation' (on the fifth or sixth level of distortion), through some form of power-seeking – maybe as a fakir or a monk, and through his own understanding achieves release, can still be drawn back by a different form of the same craving for power and become crystallised again. Some people may have to experience the entire country of a particular level of distortion, living through a variety of its possible forms, before becoming able to release themselves from its experience altogether by understanding the *principle* upon which their attraction to this kind of etheric darkness is based.

The seventh level of distortion and real etheric darkness, which is furthest away from any natural level of life and spiritual guidance and growth, is usually brought with a person into his physical life from previous existences. If he has not brought this state of 'darkness' with him in its entirety, he has come with the predisposition towards it – and more than that, for the descent into any state of distortion is never instantaneous but a slow retrogression which often takes several periods of life to accomplish, and many more to get out of again. In such a case, the physical life provides a crucial opportunity which can enable the person either to see the dangerous state of his own mind and life or to seal his condition for many 'lifetimes' to come.

The above holds true for the three lowest levels of mentality. In only very few cases do people construct these levels of mind entirely during their physical lives on earth. For the most part they are built up through a number of experiences on etheric planes and only gradually become what may best be called 'crystallised' into a certain state of mind. During this long process, and before they reach that ultimate state, enlightenment and change are always possible. It depends solely on the will of the person. Once the state of crystallisation has been reached it becomes more difficult and takes much longer – but it is never *impossible*. Enlightenment will come ultimately to everyone – not in a flash, but gradually, even to those people who have become like formations of rock in the darkness of the earth's core. No one is ever entirely beyond the reach of help from the spiritual beings engaged in the rescue of the ones who live in darkness. And if Light itself cannot penetrate to the most distant levels of distortion, the vibration of *peace* can do so, and it can bring a warmth and radiance akin to sunlight to the ones 'who sit in darkness' – when they are ready to receive it. Until that time comes they do not even know they are in darkness.

The lowest level of etheric 'reality', and the mind a person inhabits on this level, is indeed dense and hard like opaque rock – and yet the person himself presents a very different external appearance to the person on the sixth level who acts under the influence of his fanaticism. The differences are due to several factors. In the first place, all motivation derives from *outside* the person on the seventh level; there is no internal drive at all towards specific aims or goals. On every other level of distortion, a person's will is focussed on a particular aim, expressed towards a certain internal goal. Power, 'self' – even the most imaginary picture of the self, or a strong negative emotion are all points of focus which develop within the person. But on this level, where the will is at its strongest – as strong and firm and determined as rock – there is no *inner* point of focus or aim at all. There is no contact with anything internal whatsoever, no direction of any kind from within. Impetus, aim, direction of the 'life' or existence on this level derive solely from without. They are (still using the 'rock' image) reflected from the surface of the person's being. The strong will of the person at this level has, therefore, none of the consistency of aim or direction which comes alone from *inner* purpose, whatever the nature or quality of that purpose. Aims fluctuate from moment to moment, from period to period in the person's 'life' without consistency; but with each aim there is the strength of a 'rock', the will of iron to see it through. So a person on this level may present a picture of being 'all things to all men'; equally convincing in all his guises, he can deceive many people who will believe everything he says because it has the ring of authority in it. Each one will see reflected on the surface of that person his own expectations of him. The highest ideals can be *reflected* from that surface, but they cannot be carried out truly by the person because they find no resonance within him: they are not *his* ideals. Equally, his mind can reflect the greatest evils, and his will actualize them; for there is no point of contact with his own Inner Being[64] to prevent this happening.

The 'rock', into which the being of a person at this lowest level of existence has 'crystallised', has to be broken up and dissolved before he is able to return to his own natural level of life. The influence of his Inner Being can only begin to be felt by him again after the complete destruction of that rock-like being he has willed and built up as himself.

V

This teaching, about the seven levels of distortion to which any man may descend through ignorance and his own will, was first given to students of Yoga about two thousand five hundred years ago. It was given for two reasons. First of all, it was essential for people to acquire a clear picture of where failure to understand and become responsible for the direction of their own minds could lead. It was necessary for them to learn about the nature of will and to see, with unmistakable clarity, that to *will* any form of self fantasy would lead inevitably to its domination over the person; to indulge continuously in negative thinking or emotion would lead to some form of imprisonment in that emotion; and to will the craving for power, in whatever form, would cause distortions of mind and body inconceivable to anyone who had not witnessed them. The aim of imparting such knowledge was to increase the desire in individual men and women to become conscious and responsible for all aspects of their minds *now*.

The second reason for giving this teaching was that, through it, the student acquired a clearer understanding of the relationship between forms of mind and forms of etheric 'reality'. He learned to see how the states of mind which a person inhabits *inside* himself constitute in fact the world which he thinks of as existing *outside* himself. Through this knowledge the student learned to distinguish types and levels of mind in the people around him and to realise that every type or level of mind experiences a different kind of 'reality'.

This understanding becomes the starting point for a new and non-subjective way of seeing the world of human relationships and its history. It also provides a basis for a gradual realisation of the fact that although everyone *appears* to inhabit the same physical world, they really inhabit only their own form and states of mind.[65] When a person's eyes are opened to the true nature and structure of the world people inhabit, then everyone can be seen in relation to where they are internally and there is no longer any ground for the assumption that people ought to think or see or behave alike.

[1]Most contemporary books on yoga define *Pratyahara* along the lines of Patanjali (*The Yoga Aphorisms of Patanjali*) as a withdrawal or control of the senses. Patanjali speaks of a 'withdrawal of the senses ... from their proper business (so that they) are imitating ... the nature of the mind'. (II,54. Trans. by Swami Prabhavananda and Christopher Isherwood.) This means that the aim of the yogi is not merely a

withdrawal of attention at will from the messages coming in from the senses, but being able to command the senses when and how to operate. (Wood, *Yoga*, p.138. Pelican Books, 1959.)

Control of the senses in this way has never formed part of the oral teaching of Yoga. The aim was never to stop or control *in any way* the reception of impressions or to prevent their re-direction to the mind. The aim was – and is – self-knowledge: knowledge about the working of this part of man's mind, observation of its actual functioning in the individual man, and growth or extension of personal awareness.

The oral teaching has never been concerned with any 'withdrawal of the senses from their proper function' but rather with what is, in a sense, the very opposite of this statement. Its aim is to do everything to cleanse and strengthen the vehicles through which man apprehends the universe around him, for an unimpeded and accurate reception and transmission to his mind of every kind of impression, sensual and etheric. Such is the function of the *pranayama* exercises. An entirely new stage is begun by a man after the development of his 'new' will, when objective experience and the reception of objective reality begin to become possible. But every new stage reached by a man in the course of his spiritual evolution depends on the correct and proper functioning of every aspect of his being, according to its inherent nature. No true growth can proceed from a distortion of any part of a man's nature. A 'withdrawal of the senses from their proper function' would lead to such a distortion (or perversion) and create an obstacle to real spiritual development.

In the same way, this oral teaching has never encouraged 'the senses to imitate the mind of man', as is obvious from all that is written above. For the senses *are* the mind of man, or rather form a large and coherent part of its structure which takes in every vibration which he receives from his environment.

[2]The Enneagram Triangle, which has already been discussed above, stands for the totality of man's mind. Point 3 on it stands for this passive sense organ which receives everything coming into the man's mind from outside his own etheric body.

[3]This mental organ of the senses has nothing to do with the *registering* of impressions but only with receiving them in a certain way, according to its nature and development. The impressions which are *only* registered and not actually received do not remain long but gradually fade and leave no memory-trace. So, also, the *true* nature of impressions does not remain with a person but only that particular form of them in which they are received by his mind or his own mental sense organ.

[4]Buddhism provides an image of the person who, having achieved 'en-lightenment' beyond the etheric sphere, nevertheless returns to that sphere to help with the redemption of all mankind and remains in that sphere until all mankind is regenerated. This is the Boddhisattwa.

[5]I.e., no form of creation.

[6]Will also enters into the creation of all subjective reality but not consciously, and only insofar as it initiates or calls into action the process of creation.

[7]Cultures or societies are usually seen to have a natural rhythm of growth, maturity, and decay and possible regeneration.

[8]There are many recorded experiences of quite ordinary people as well as of mystics in which this 'jump' in mental/etheric level is clearly illustrated (See, for example, F.C. Happold's *Mysticism*, Pelican Books, 1963). A person in whom this happens suddenly finds himself on another plane of reality where he experiences a mundane happening in an entirely new way, or an everyday object is unexpectedly transformed in appearance, or heretofor, unrelated objects or ideas come together to form a coherent and meaningful pattern. What has in fact happened is that the person experiences another and higher mental level which opens out onto another etheric level of reality. Wherever he is, in his thoughts and in his external

environment, at the moment of this happening, is transformed for him because of the mental state through which he experiences it. The same 'things' exist as before – the same trees, grass, landscape; the same thoughts, ideas, relationships – but the reality-tone of everything is different. The person experiences a new level of the etheric reality of everything around and within him. Some of the mental structure and limitation of the level of mind he usually inhabits no longer exist on the higher level and so the reality he sees is 'new', although it is related to the previous one.

[9]The movement 'downward' is *never* back to a previous level in the etheric growth pattern through which a person has evolved, but *always* into one of the seven forms of distortion or perversion, depending entirely upon the mental state and will of the individual concerned.

[10]Everyone is born into that form of society which most nearly corresponds to the nature, structure, and stage of his own mind.

[11]One of the principle aims of practical Yoga teaching is to re-connect with these memory-traces, which is possible through the *kundalini sense*.

[12]This applies to both Western and Eastern people, for even those born into cultures that use such terms as karma or reincarnation to explain life do not find ready access to their own personal memory-traces.

[13]It is the structure of mind of people on a certain level – that is, on a certain level of etheric or mental reality – which gives this interpretation to their intimations of previous existence. It is from this same etheric level that the theory of reincarnation was evolved and to which it exclusively belongs.

[14]With the exception of certain rare experiences of extended reality, when a person may experience momentarily on a higher level. Usually, however, such experiences are based on an extended awareness of the level he already inhabits.

[15]This is the same as the situation on the physical earth, where people with very different qualities of being or levels of mentality can live side by side yet unconscious of the *essential* differences which separate them.

[16]Requests, desires, inclinations *harmful* to the person or to others – *if persevered in* – draw that person to its fulfilment on one of the seven lower levels.

[17]'Paradise' of every form and shape is an expression of man's highest conception of possession, of that ambience in which he would most like to live or experience himself: the Heaven of heavens, the 'floating life' ...

[18]Desire for the tangible or for a material result finds a response more easily on the etheric plane than on the physical plane.

[19]No 'consciousness of change' but certainly an increase in consciousness beyond that which exists among the inhabitants of the first etheric level, for growth in consciousness is one of the primary characteristics of man's evolution.

[20]'Creative' activity, in which the person is solely concerned with *self* expression, is not necessarily creative at all. It may derive from the desire in the person to *have* something for himself – possibly a sense of importance or adulation from others or the experience of sensationalising – and belongs to the first level of etheric reality, or the Summerland. It could be the expression of someone on a *lower* etheric level. True creativity can only begin when the desire to communicate to others has been born in the person.

[21]They do not have anything to do with people who are engaged in lives on the *physical* plane, for they are ministered to by people from a higher etheric level.

[22]Although people on the second etheric level *minister to* new arrivals in the Summerland, they are not responsible for the *direction* or organisation of this ministration. They carry out orders, as would a nursing staff, given by people from a higher level of consciousness and understanding who know the needs of each new arrival and have prepared the structure necessary for their rehabilitation.

[23]This is one of the laws which operates on all the etheric levels through which man evolves, that no one is allowed to be harmed in any way. A person may harm himself but never another person against his will. This means that each person's spiritual growth is protected absolutely from interference or harm by another. Through the person's own free will alone can his downfall or distraction or distortion come about. The desire to pursue the self will, even to the point of harming others, can cause that person to descend to a lower level. The exercise of the self will on any one of these first four etheric levels, to the detriment of others and in sole pursuit of self interest, can cause the person to 'fall' to a lower level. A person can fall in many ways and many times.

[24]*All* people undertaking work on the earth through physical mediums are either on the second etheric level or else on one of the 'lower' planes. Such work is undertaken by the free will of the individual concerned. It could never belong to or proceed from the third etheric level where the dangers of this kind of work are understood; for mediumistic work generally causes more harm than good overall to the people involved, and can cause serious distortion to the beings of people who are in physical bodies.

[25]He may be precipitate and commence this work from his self will before he is properly prepared for it through his own spiritual evolution and so cause more harm than good to others and delay or side-track his own growth of being.

[26]The personal self is the habitual or traditional 'self', composed during the long ages of different experiences, built up and modified over aeons of time, in which the person's feeling of identity is centred. It is based as much on what it *excludes* as on what it *includes*.

[27]The personal self will is expanded here to its uppermost limit, reaching out to include all who are in need. It is nonetheless still this self will from which the desire to be of service springs; the totally new feeling of *concern* – awakened in the Heart Centre – arises only after this desire of the self will to be of service has reached its uttermost limit.

[28]'Law' means two things here. It refers to a non-personal force – although originally created by persons – which operates on all the higher etheric levels automatically to protect all life from harm. It also refers to the sequence of events or occurrences which follow, again automatically, from people's actions. In this case, the operation of the Law of Protection draws into simultaneous operation the Law of Affinities through which the person either suffers the results of which he is the cause or else is attracted to a lower sphere where his distortion may be expressed freely.

[29]It does not operate automatically on the physical plane.

[30]Called by many people the Guardian Angel. Sometimes people are 'chosen' or asked to perform this mission by someone from a higher level or stage than themselves; in other cases, people make their own decisions to accompany someone on earth from a sense of responsibility towards that person.

[31]Not all people are born onto the earth from those levels on which alone spiritual evolution is possible. Approximately forty per cent of all people born onto the physical earth in the twentieth century have been born from one of the lower spheres, with some form of mental distortion.

[32]Most people have only one spiritual companion or Guardian Angel, although some people have more than one at certain times when they have crucial tasks to perform, for example, through their positions in society, or have taken certain responsibilities of a personal or spiritual nature upon themselves.

[33]All people born before their time from the Summerland or one of the higher levels have some affinity with a lower level or they would not have been born prematurely. They have all spent time on a lower level and it is through their connections with it that they are born before their time. This applies to only about twenty-five per cent of

the people born before their time, for the majority of such people are born from one of the lower levels of distortion.

[34]They may have around them invisible companions from the lower levels to whom they are attracted and may not be in a state where they could receive spiritual guidance – or act upon it if they could receive it. They are not usually concerned with spiritual growth, so a spiritual guide would be wasting his time. But should a change come about in their beings, in the course of their physical lives, a spiritual companion would at once be attracted to them.

[35]The state of withdrawal into contemplation means withdrawal from the person's own life, exclusion of his responsibilities, limitation; it represents, *at every stage*, a retrogression, and all techniques or ideologies that encourage it are destructive of the very essence of human nature and purpose.

[36]The *reflective mind* is the fourteenth.

[37]The dimensions of *conscious awareness* are identical with those of the person's mind; in this sense, *consciousness* is synonymous with *mind*. However, a person's awareness can extend beyond consciousness into the penumbra of his mind to pick up, in a shadowy way, impressions which it cannot accept consciously or which do not completely fit into his present mental structure. Some of these may come from stages of experience through which he has passed in previous forms of existence.

[38]The 'working back' is different with each person and relates solely to his own state and the kind or degree of distortion into which he has entered. It has to do with re-tracing his own steps back to the state and condition of spiritual aliveness from which his distortion originally began. It does not involve a 'journey' through any other forms of distortion or levels of lesser 'darkness', for these are not relevant to his pattern of life at that time.

[39]On the first and second levels the forms of attachment and distortion are 'real' only to the person himself and therefore constitute *subjective reality*.

[40]But on all the other levels a person's conscience can still reach his conscious mind and keep him open to the ministrations and help with which he is always surrounded.

[41]His experiences are not *wholly* limited by it.

[42]If the person is living on the physical plane, the true nature of his mentality and the structure of his being are not readily apparent to those about him. The aspects which are observable are usually attributed to extraneous causes.

[43]This possibility of descent to a still lower level does not exist on any of the other levels.

[44]Resentment is always involved but it is not always the central feature or cause of this structure of negative emotion; there is always a relationship on which the person is 'hung up' and which has crystallised in its negative form, and thus affects the total life of the person.

[45]Only ten per cent of those who incarnate from this second lower level are able to retrace their steps, to their natural level of being, while in a physical body.

[46]The illness of *autism*, which has only been fully identified in recent years – and appears to be on the increase, is an illness or distortion of *will*. Children born in the state of autism are often intelligent although they present a picture of withdrawal and wilful refusal to relate. The causes always lie in previous forms of existence, for they are the most serious manifestations of that form of distortion in the will which structures the minds of all people on this second lower level. *Autism* represents the worst state of entropy into which a person can get, and there is only the rare possibility of real change during a physical lifetime. The will usually remains at least partially paralysed while the person is still in a physical body.

[47]They can 'injure' but not do violence to or affect permanently the mind of another person. If a person's mind includes doing violence to others, he inhabits not the third but the *fifth* lower level.

[48]This is in contrast with the second level, where it is only with great difficulty that a person is able to become free from his particular negative and introverted mental state during a physical life on earth.

[49]To begin with people enter a place only temporarily as they experience *passing* states of envy, desire, frustration; but they can come to *inhabit* such places for increasingly longer periods of time.

[50]All the lower levels were created – and are still being created – by people on the lowest levels of distortion and darkness. The *places* which they create can be entered by anyone, anywhere on the first four levels of the etheric sphere – by people in physical as well as in etheric bodies – who allows that form of distortion to dominate his mind which corresponds to the outer *place*. These places have *objective* existence. Although distorted beings can create such places, they are not able to interfere with anyone – beyond their dimensions. Their power and influence belong only to their own, 'self' created spheres; their power extends only to those people who allow it entrance by their own distortion or disharmony.

[51]All forms of sexual perversion or deviation belong to this level unless they do violence to others, in which case they belong to the next lower or fifth level.

[52]All *true* homosexuality belongs to this level or place of being.

[53]'Athletic exploitation' of the physical body through exaggerated or one-sided training and exercise.

[54]'Lasting', that is, throughout the physical life into the etheric form of existence.

[55]All that is said here, with regard to the fourth lower level, applies equally to the fifth level of distortion.

[56]*Violence* is a distortion of the natural power inherent in will.

[57]Some teachers in various cults or 'esoteric' groups seek to destroy the naturally spontaneous creative essence of life in those whom they try to subvert to their particular doctrine; and sometimes those who organise extremist groups 'dedicated' to one cause or another belong to the fifth level of distortion.

[58]That is, true *schizophrenie*. But people are often labelled schizophrenic who are not so in the true meaning of the word, or only partially so, but may have certain of its characteristics such as rigid compartmentalisation of mind or certain forms of violence of which they are unaware.

[59]This construction always takes place on etheric planes. The formation of the schizophrenic mind is always completed on these planes and never on the physical plane; so the person with a truly schizoid mind brings it with him into physical life.

[60]This is a schizophrenic *being* not merely a 'personality', for it represents an essential division within the person which reflects the nature of that person. It also has the quality of *permanence* in him until he reaches the point where he is willing and prepared to be healed.

[61]The schizophrenic can be helped and made whole during his physical life – but never by anyone in the 'normal' compartment of his life. Family and friends, if they are in this normal compartment, can never help him successfully – nor can the usual forms of professional assistance. He can only be helped by someone from within his own form of perversion: one of his own victims or a fellow prisoner – should he be committed to prison – or another schizophrenic in whom the compartmentalisation is breaking down and who is on the way to being healed. This is a law of healing: Only someone who has suffered the same illness can be used to help another. Another law is that at a certain stage in the healing process of a person, he must give help to another sufferer before healing can proceed in himself.

[62]At least, so far as current thinking is concerned. In fact, however, *mind* and *place* are the same thing in real terms, for every person truly inhabits the mind he has created for himself.

[63]The first and second levels of distortion are the only ones which have a certain connection with one another.

[64]His Inner Being contains all he has experienced and learned in the past and acquired by way of understanding, which could restrain him from evil.

[65]Marked dissimilarities between people are due to *real* differences in their minds and etheric levels of being. Antagonisms in human life arise, in large part, from an assumption of similarity and equality that is based on ignorance of the nature of etheric reality and the different levels of mind and being.

CHAPTER FIVE

DHARANA, DHYANA, SAMADHI

The teaching of Yoga as it was originally taught, and as it has been given to students orally over a period of nearly six thousand years, was designed to lead people to the stage of Pratyahara. Only vague indications were given as to the pattern of human growth and evolution beyond that stage. The primary aim of Yoga was the right formation of *mind* which would lead men to acquire those experiences best suited to them individually, in their own unique patterns of growth. The right formation of mind in each person would also make of it an instrument which he could ultimately use in the highest degree of service to others on the third and fourth etheric levels. The stage of Pratyahara corresponds in most respects to the fourth level of etheric reality or mind, which is the level of those who have achieved or are achieving that advanced stage in their evolution where they are able to be responsible spiritually for other people as well as themselves. This Yoga teaching has essentially to do with the perfection of the personal self and with its growth from the most primitive forms of self, and the expressions of will based on like/dislike, through every stage of self expression to the ultimate stage of self expression in the service of others.

The entrance into a person of an entirely new element, around which forms in time a new centre of gravity, is a stage which lay on the furthermost frontier of this ancient Yoga teaching. The commencement of non-personal[1] Caring or Concern in a person, focussed in his Heart Centre, was a very distant prospect for most men on earth at that time, nearly six thousand years ago. Very few people were at a point in their own individual evolutions where teaching on this subject would have had relevancy; it could have been at most abstract or theoretical – and the purpose of Yoga is to provide useful instruction to help people where they *are* in their own beings. Most of the early teachers of Yoga had evolved only up to the fourth level, although some were on the fifth etheric level; but none had evolved beyond that stage. Their knowledge of later stages and further goals was therefore incomplete. Some of the knowledge which they, in fact, possessed was given to their students as a vague outline of distant stages; but they exercised selectivity and knowledge was withheld which could have caused harm or distortion through misunderstanding. It was not until several thousand years later that this part of the teaching was given more fully;[2] by that time the need was greater, for there were more human beings incarnate on earth who could absorb knowledge about the later stages in their etheric evolution.

In some – but not all – respects, the stage of Pratyahara corresponds to the fourth level of etheric reality; similarly, the stages of *Dharana, Dhyana*, and *Samadhi* correspond in many respects to the fifth, sixth, and seventh etheric levels.

The Old Sanskrit word *As* (as in *As-ana*) stands for the 'personal' mind, which is the entire mind of a man at the second and third stages,[3] centred around a 'personal self'. The mind denoted by *As* includes all structures of mind that grow out of different images of 'self' formed by like, dislike, desire; and all desires for and forms of self expression, including the structure of mind which develops out of the desire to be of service to others. The exercises for a man at this stage are concerned with making his mind more flexible (*ana*). *As-ana* describes the fullest possible development of a man's *As* (personal mind), which means ultimately not only flexibility but sensitivity and responsiveness to direction – the direction of his own evolution. All change of mind depends upon these three things.

The personal mind or *As* is dominant in man up to and including the fourth etheric level; but at that level another element enters in to provide a new growing point from which, in time, a new mind will evolve. Before the new mind can take form, however, a struggle develops in the man between the two aspects of mind, the personal (or old mind, or *As*) and the non-personal (or sense of Concern or Caring);[4] out of this struggle comes the desire to search for God. This desire, this single will, focussed solely on the search for God, develops in the person a single or one-pointed mind.[5] In Old Sanskrit, this one-pointed mind was called *Dhar*.

The next stage, or step, in man's evolution is called *Dharana* and has to do with the greatest possible development of his single, focussed mind which has become concentrated through his will to find God. In teachings that developed subsequently to the original oral teaching, *Dharana* has been defined as 'concentration', which, in a sense, correctly denotes the purpose of the work and exercises performed at this point in man's evolution. But the work of concentration must be understood in relation to *Dhar*: the mind of man at this stage or level in his evolution; for, otherwise, the exercises would at best be irrelevant to his needs and, at worst, distort the pattern of his growth. When the knowledge about man's evolution, and the pattern of stages through which he evolves, became lost, so the stage called *Dharana* was seen merely as an 'aspect' of Yoga practices and the exercises in 'concentration' were dissociated from their original aim or altered.

In fact, the teaching about *Dharana* is teaching about the work which takes place on the fifth etheric level, where the person's whole being is centred on his search for God. It means, in essence, learning to use the single-focussed mind with infinite sensitivity and responsiveness to turn in upon itself and seek through all previous experiences for God. This is an enormous task, for it involves not only the concentrated search through the mind itself and all previous experiences which the person has had, but a re-visiting of places and people out of which those experiences arose. This task can take several thousand 'years' of time, while the work is being pursued on various etheric planes.

The Old Sanskrit word *ana* is used in relation to three different stages, *As-ana, Dhar-ana*, and *Dhy-ana*. In each of these three stages it refers to the perfection of the particular kind of *mind* which belongs to the respective stage. In the first case, it has to do with the growth and development of the personal mind. In the second case, *ana* is concerned with the fullest possible development of the mind denoted as *Dhar*, which means a focussing upon itself and the development of complete awareness of every experience which has gone into its formation. At this stage the word *ana* means the learning of total concentration and inner awareness *in order that the mind may become completely conscious of itself and of all that has gone into its composition and structuring*. This is the aim of the stage or level of man's evolution called *Dharana*.

At the third stage, *Dhyana*, the word *ana* is used to denote the development of Objective Mind in man.

The word *ana* is not a noun, which stands for a state already acquired or developed, but a verb denoting activity and the efforts necessary to become aware, or more sensitive, or to stay awake to purpose and direction. It implies, therefore, the making of special kinds of effort – not the efforts necessitated by a man's physical life on earth or called forth by his life on etheric planes, but *extra* effort: effort needed to go against a tendency to drift which exists in every man on both the etheric and physical planes. Growth of being at every stage depends upon this extra effort signified by the word *ana*; and consistent effort is required to achieve those attributes which belong, in differing degrees and qualities, to the three different kinds of mind,[6] namely, flexibility, sensitivity, responsiveness to direction – and, above all, the effort needed to stay 'awake'.

The tendency to drift exists in all etheric life; it is a tendency to entropy, for it is impossible to drift 'upwards'. Growth in all etheric life – whether plant or animal or man – requires effort, the effort of pushing beyond the limits of the state or condition already achieved, whatever that might be. It is will – the Divine Will in its own particular and appropriate form – that activates the seed so that the seed-state may be transcended and plant-life formed. So it is with man. In man, the tendency to entropy belongs to the nature of his mind; the substance of mind naturally recedes, draws together, becomes passive, if it is not acted upon by the person's will. The achievement of every new state or condition of mind, the working through of every experience a man enters into in order to acquire understanding, and the creation of every facet in his mind out of this understanding are the result of continuous effort of will.

Only after a certain stage has been reached, at the end of the fourth etheric level, when a man's mind has been completely formed with regard to its basic structure of personal experience,[7] is a point of stability attained which is permanent for him. At this point, his mind becomes 'fixed' at the outermost limits of expansion *possible for him*, and from this point it can no longer draw back or recede. This is the ultimate achievement of that stage denoted by the word *Asana*. Beyond that stage, renewed effort is required for man as he works within and towards the fulfilment of the stage denoted as *Dharana*. And beyond that again, after it has achieved its perfection – after the man's mind has clarified as a many-facetted crystal, there is the next – and final – stage of *Dhyana* in which his efforts are focussed on the cleansing and polishing of each crystal for the achievement of Objective Mind. At each of these succeeding stages, the tendency to entropy is still an integral part of his mind and he can still drift back to what had become fixed in him at the previous stage, which is the foundation for his renewed efforts. Each new stage or formation of mind may take hundreds, or even thousands, of years to accomplish – especially if the person allows himself to drift and his mind to diminish.

When a student reaches the stage of *Dharana* his life doesn't necessarily alter in any external sense. He doesn't literally move to a new country or take on a new job – whether on a physical or etheric plane; nor is it necessary for him to relinquish his physical or etheric life *as it is* and retire from the world he inhabits so as to pursue undisturbed exercises in 'concentration'. All exercises connected with *Dharana* are designed to facilitate the mind's concentration upon its inward journey and search, but they are performed – or undertaken – within the person's life of *outer activity*.[8] All change takes place where he is – and this is true for every stage – and is invisible to those around him. For a person who has already passed out of a physical body and is engaged in tasks relevant to the fourth etheric level, the stage of *Dharana* and its exercises do not imply necessarily – or immediately – another task or another 'country'. All movement and all changes are *internal* to begin with, that is, changes in the *ground* of the person's thinking, seeing, acting; they are only gradually reflected in the whole life of the person.

Dharana means a stage or level in man's spiritual evolution or pattern of growth; it also refers to the activity or work or efforts of a man at this stage to achieve that sensitivity, responsiveness, awareness of mind – and the kind of mind which the word *Dhar* denotes. At the end of this stage, man's search for God becomes transformed into a search for Truth. And the Truth to which he becomes receptive is the Truth about himself: his own mind, his own being. At the conclusion of this stage a man is in full possession of self-knowledge; he has achieved complete awareness of himself and of all the experiences which, over aeons of time, have contributed to the growth of his etheric mind.

The next stage begins with the state reached by the previous one, which is the mind filled with the light of self-awareness and radiating Truth about its own nature. *Dhyana* corresponds in most respects to the sixth level of reality and is concerned with perfecting the mind so that it is able to reflect Objective Truth, that is, Truth about the spheres in which a man has his being and that comprise all etheric life to which he is related and for which he has any responsibility.

The Old Sanskrit word *Dhy*, or *Dhi*, means the perfected etheric mind, which is a mind cleansed in each aspect and every 'crystal-face' so that it is capable of the perfect reflection of all etheric life. The completed mind, or *Dhar*, is structured like a crystal of many faces, each of whose facets was formed by a seminal experience in the ages-long life history of the particular man. Each crystal-face in his mind is completely structured by the time he has reached the end of the fifth stage and represents, or symbolises, the *kind* of experience which originally produced it. By the end of this fifth stage, the person has learned the Truth about the nature of every experience he has undergone leading to an understanding of its essence and the formation of a corresponding structure in his own mind. At the sixth stage, the final perfecting of this mind consists in his learning to use each facet to reflect accurately, or truthfully, any similar experience within his own orbit of relationships (which may extend to every point in the etheric world through which he has himself evolved). The perfected etheric mind, or *Dhy*, in a man is an instrument capable of reflecting Objective Truth.

The self-knowledge achieved at the fifth stage, or *Dharana*, does not lead the person to an understanding of the *essence* of each experience which underlies the formation of every facet of his mind; for that essence is revealed only at the sixth level when he begins to use his mind as an instrument of perception for the understanding of others. Then, only, is this essence slowly distilled after the 'personal' elements have become recognisable to him. The person then begins to see the causes which produced the particular experience, the etheric level of reality to which it belongs, and the principles involved in its resolution. As his understanding grows, so the facet of mind which a particular experience formed in him is cleansed and becomes gradually capable of reflecting all other similar experiences objectively.[9] This is the way in which the mind is cleansed. It is not primarily an interior process, concentrated inwards as at the stage of *Dharana*, with its focus on the search for God; but it is a process based on certain forms of *meditation* and related practices in awareness which extend *outwards* to include, in time, the entire 'universe' of a man, which is the sum of all his relationships and experiences. These exercises in meditation do not concentrate upon *self* awareness, that is, awareness of what has already been formed in the person's mind, but are a way of teaching him to *use* the different facets of his mind to perceive the exact nature and needs of human, animal, and plant life about him. The word 'exact' is important, for the exercises teach a man to use his mind as a precision instrument for the perception of Objective Truth. This is the way in which each facet of his mind is cleansed, through learning to use it as a precision tool and distinguishing the elements in it which are subjective or 'personal' to himself; for a mental facet can only reflect Truth when the person is aware of all its subjective aspects. Conversely, no mental facet can be cleansed of its personal elements until the individual has reached the stage where he truly seeks to use it as a mirror to reflect someone else's need. For example, if he tries to use a facet of his own mind – which was formed through the experience of a certain kind of suffering – to understand the nature of another person's suffering and learn what help (if any) he can give, so its objective structure and the principles on which his experience was based clarify and are distinguishable from the subjective elements, which cannot reflect Truth at all.

The desire for Truth is the principal characteristic of someone at the sixth level of reality, and it is this desire for Truth which provides the strongest motive force for the cleansing of every facet of mind.

So long as a man fails to recognise the subjective elements in his own mind, he may be aware of many of the needs of people around him but his mind will not be an accurate instrument for the precise registering of the nature of these needs. Even more important, his mind will be incapable of registering *what is spiritually possible* for other people. At every stage in human evolution, even in the Summerland, the human mind is capable of registering, and identifying, some vibrations in other people which are akin to itself. A man who has a certain kind of like or desire can often pick up a similar like or desire in other people. In fact, it is *through* the very characteristics in his own mind, whatever its nature or level of reality, that he is able to register and identify these same characteristics in others. But it is only at the sixth etheric level, that the mind in its ultimate stage of development becomes able to register human *potential.* To have a vision of another person's potential means being able to perceive where that person is in his own pattern of evolution and in what direction the next possible stage in his development lies. This vision is more important than being able to perceive the person's difficulties, needs, or the obstacles which stand in the way of his development. Only at this sixth level, can a man learn to know what is *right* for the other person and so avoid the risk of causing distortion to his being or diverting him from his true direction or damaging his will, all of which possibilities exist so long as the man's mind contains unrecognised subjective elements. No real help can be given until his mind is capable of a true vision of the other person's potential as well as of his need.

The mind of the man at the sixth level of reality is extended to its greatest possible extent and is in touch with every part of the etheric world through which it has personally evolved, including various forms of animal and plant life. Therefore, the exercises which belong to this stage of *Dhyana* have nothing to do with mind-extension, for that is no longer necessary; they are concerned with learning to discern the underlying nature of the world and the truth which exists in all relationships and forms of expression. They are concerned with teaching the mind to perceive Truth in all things. The exercises may be described as the practice of certain forms of *meditation* whose aim is to enable the nature of a certain object or relationship to be reflected truthfully by the mind and comprehended accurately by the person's consciousness.

These exercises in meditation are practised in the midst of the person's ordinary activity, whatever that might be – whether on the physical or the etheric plane – and never in total isolation from the person's life of external relationships. In general the *Dhyana* exercises concern mental activity of a two-fold nature. Both parts relate to the central activity of this stage, which is learning to understand the true nature of a certain person, object, or relationship. The first exercise has to do with the person identifying all the 'personal' elements in the particular facet of his own mind through which he is endeavouring to perceive an object or relationship. The second exercise consists in the person projecting his own consciousness into the particular object so that he receives *direct knowledge* of its nature from within. These are two quite distinct and separate exercises, involving different kinds of mental activity, both of which, in various forms, are essential to the work of this stage and fundamental to the reception of every kind of Objective Knowledge whether it relates to another person, the operation of an etheric principle or law, the nature of an animal, or the essential vibration of a certain plant.

Other exercises are also used at this stage as training in the extension of consciousness, so that a pattern may be laid down for its use in actual situations. One of these exercises consists in selecting three different *kinds* of object for meditation, for example, a particular plant, an animal, and a person. The objects must always be specific and known to the meditator, and not generalised abstractions. He visualises each object in turn with his Creative Imagination and extends his consciousness into it, moving about in each image and occupying it as fully as possible. Each image is 'inhabited' in this way for approximately eight minutes; the whole exercise takes about thirty minutes. To become truly effective it should be repeated each day at the same time, the same three images used on three consecutive days before they are replaced with three new ones.

Another exercise, which forms part of this stage of *Dhyana*, has to do with a man learning to place his consciousness in the Head Centre and receive increased inspiration, direction, and knowledge through it. This exercise must *never* be attempted 'abstractly' or repeated regularly; it is one which should only be practised in relation to a particular need or situation. The person must first of all *need* to seek direction of a certain kind or to be given knowledge to increase his understanding of a particular situation. In time, as the Head Centre is put increasingly to its proper use, so the person's own receptivity grows and he becomes more and more able to receive from a level of knowledge which can only be transmitted in this way.

In many respects the two kinds of exercise overlap. Where the person seeks a deeper understanding of some relationship or situation, he may meditate upon it by projecting his consciousness into the image he has visualised of it; or he may, by concentrating upon the Head Centre, receive knowledge of a kind which goes beyond what his consciousness at any one time is able to comprehend; or he may use both exercises.

These two kinds of exercise appear simple and therefore accessible to anyone, at any stage in his pattern of evolution. In fact, they belong *only* to the stage of *Dhyana*. They must not be undertaken at any other stage, before all the work and exercises appropriate to the preceding stages have been gone through and the person has evolved to the sixth etheric level. For it is only at this point that the transfer of a man's centre of gravity (or feeling of 'I') finally takes place from the Sex Centre to his real etheric being and its manifestation through the three upper centres. Only after this change in his centre of gravity is complete can it be said that the man has finally evolved beyond the sphere of his personal self. While this transfer is taking place, work is going on simultaneously in his mind of identifying the subjective or 'personal' elements which prevent the facets in his mind from reflecting Objective Knowledge. Until this work is complete and the mind of the man has been cleansed of all that links it subconsciously with the personal self, and until his feeling of 'I' is no longer influenced in any degree at all by the Sex Centre and its desire for power, these exercises must not be undertaken. The danger from attempting to perform spiritual exercises out of their proper context lies in the distortion they can cause in the growth-pattern of the individual. If the *Dhyana* exercises in meditation were attempted at an earlier stage, they would increase the personal or subjective attributes of mind and the man's own identification with these attributes, making far more difficult the mind's eventual cleansing. Furthermore, the knowledge received through the practice of these exercises at an earlier stage would not be Objective Knowledge for it would be distorted by the mind of the person performing them. Objective Knowledge can only be obtained if they are practised in their right context. Great danger could also accrue to other people if the person imagined he was able to receive Truth about people, relationships, or situations before he could in fact do so.

A man who reaches this sixth etheric level during his physical lifetime on earth will find that certain characteristics or attributes of mind – which do not seem 'personal' to him, insofar as they do not describe his feeling of himself, and yet form part of his mental structure – never seem to fade away completely. In fact, they are capable of being re-activated as long as the person inhabits a physical body. This can cause a certain amount of distress until he realises that these are part of the social-cultural context in which he developed physically, and from which he 'acquired' them, and that they belong to the 'mind' of the culture rather than to his own mind. They form part of his own mind only through his participation in the cultural mind. When he becomes aware of them, they need no longer form an *integral* part of his own mind; nevertheless, they do not fade away entirely so long as he is living a physical life.

These exercises which are related to the stage of *Dhyana* constitute the hub of a new life. They are not exercises to be learned or practised for a time and then dropped. They form the basis not only for a new way of thinking and using the mind, but they actually *constitute* a new mind which opens out into a new kind of life, whether a man is on the physical or the etheric plane. The mind becomes a mirror which truly reflects the entire world in which that man lives:

all levels of etheric reality and all orders and forms of reality which belong to his life-history. It is unlike the experience of empathy which existed at an earlier stage and in which the person retained his own barriers, his careful and clearly-felt definitions of himself. In 'empathy' there is both 'self' and 'other' as two completely separated entities. Now, as he evolves through this stage of *Dhyana*, there is no fear of losing the self, for this 'self' no longer exists but has been entirely replaced by another self. His consciousness is freed from that former self and the fear of losing it and so it can move and experience wherever his will directs it.

When the person has reached this point where his mind is wholly cleansed and able to reflect Truth with every separate facet and the will is able to extend its consciousness and so enter into every person, object, or situation reflected by the mind, then the person has entered the last and final etheric stage of *Samadhi*.

The word *S-ama-dhi* is a composite word, built up of three separate elements whose meanings fully describe the nature and work of this final etheric stage. *Dhi* means the same as *dhy*: that is, the complete etheric mind, with its fully cleansed facets, capable of reflecting every aspect of etheric life through which the person has previously evolved over long aeons of time. The letter *S* is an Old Sanskrit symbol for the other essential and irreducible body of man,[10] called his 'long body'. The long body of a man is made up of *all* etheric life for which he is personally responsible, but consists primarily of certain essential relationships to other people which have been formed throughout his own evolution through many different stages. These relationships are not revealed as to their essential nature until the man reaches the sixth etheric level. Until that time, he will often consider many relationships important which are not so and relationships that belong to his long body he may overlook altogether. This 'long body', when it becomes fully formed and visible to the man, is seen as a 'body' of people related not to one another but solely to himself and for whose spiritual evolution he is ultimately responsible.

The word or symbol *ama* stands between the *S* and the *dhi* and denotes something akin to meditation or awareness; but *ama* means more than 'awareness'. Many different practices of meditation or awareness have accompanied the person through every stage in his evolution, from the latter part of the second etheric level onwards, all of which have had to do with the growth and extension of his mind – the mind of each stage in turn. Only latterly and to a lesser degree has meditation been concerned with the development of will. All the practices of meditation have had to do more with the development of the *passive* than the *active* part of man, that is, with the development of his mind as an instrument of perception or receptivity. At this ultimate stage in man's etheric evolution, however, *ama* does not refer to the development of the *passive* part of man's nature – for his etheric mind has already reached its final state of perfection – but to the evolution of the *active* part of his being, which is his will.

This development of will is expressed in two ways. First of all, the will develops the potential expressed in the image of the Divine Will through learning to use the Creative Imagination to its full capacity actually to create life; and, secondly, it grows into its complete sense of responsibility towards use of the etheric mind (*dhi*) and evolution of the people who make up his 'long body' (*S*).

There are two stages in the development of a man's will on this seventh etheric level. At the first stage, the will learns to act wholly from Truth; Truth becomes the sole motive from which the man's actions spring. At the second stage in this evolution of will, it becomes wholly inspired by Caring or Concern.

The symbol *ama* faces in both directions, standing above the man's two different 'bodies' (*dhi* and *S*) as the responsible, creative, and Caring will – at the fullest extension of its evolution within the etheric spheres known to man. Beyond these spheres lies the Unknown. At some distant point this Unknown will draw the man's will onwards, but for the moment he rests in the achievement of that evolutionary path upon which he set out at the dawn of his consciousness manifold aeons before.

[1]Meaning, not self-oriented – rather than impersonal.

[2]'The Fulfilment of Yoga in the Higher Teaching' was given nearly four thousand years later.

[3]See Chapter Four, Pratyahara, III, pp. 173-4.

[4]In fact, there is only *one* mind, but many stages of it. At this stage, when a new centre of focus for mind is being formed, from which a transformed mind can evolve, there *appear* to be two separate minds.

[5]Both centres of gravity, the Sex Centre and the point of Caring in the Heart Centre, are focussed temporarily for this stage on the single aim or purpose expressed in the man's search for God.

[6]That is, *As*, *Dhar*, and *Dhy*.

[7]After that point, a man does not need – or seek for – new personal experience but re-works the structure of experience he has already acquired from the point of view of his search for God. At the next, or sixth, etheric level he again works through his structure of experience and mind in order to create the ultimate etheric state, or Objective Mind, in himself.

[8]At *every* stage in man's evolution, whether he is on the physical plane or on an etheric plane, *outer* activity of some kind is an integral part of his existence.

[9]The person's understanding of a particular experience – formed into a specific facet of mind – remains with him permanently after all the 'personal' elements in the experience have disappeared altogether from his memory.

[10]The first 'essential and irreducible body' of man is his complete etheric mind or *dhi*. All other 'bodies' which he possesses, or sees, or thinks he possesses, are reflections or expressions of his etheric mind. Even his physical body is a temporary expression of and vehicle for his etheric mind (and his will) to experience through. The person's *will* does not in itself constitute a body.